As *Stand Tall* goes to press, the information it contains is current and up-to-date. Future editions will cover newer developments. Between editions, you may want a way to stay in touch with what is going on, as research continues, new discoveries are made, and new prevention and treatment drugs are developed.

The National Osteoporosis Foundation (NOF) can be your link to new information. NOF is America's only non-profit voluntary health organization dedicated to reducing the widespread prevalence of osteoporosis through programs of research, education and advocacy.

For information on NOF's quarterly newsletter or to contact its Patient Information Center, write to 1150 17th Street, NW, Washington, DC 20036 or call them at (202) 223-2226.

STAND TALL!

Every Woman's Guide to
PREVENTING AND TREATING OSTEOPOROSIS

Second Edition

Morris Notelovitz, MD, PhD
with Marsha Ware, MD
and Diana Tonnessen

Physical Therapy Consultant
Sara Meeks, PT, GCS

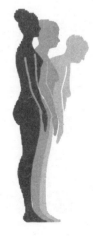

 TRIAD PUBLISHING COMPANY   GAINESVILLE, FLORIDA

Library of Congress Cataloging-in-Publication Data
Notelovitz, Morris
    Stand tall!   every woman's guide to preventing and treating
  osteoporosis / Morris Notelovitz, with Marsha Ware and Diana
  Tonnessen : physical therapy consultant, Sara Meeks. -- 2nd ed.
        p.   cm.
    Includes bibliographical references and index.
    ISBN 0-937404-38-1 (hc)
    1. Osteoporosis in women.   2. Osteoporosis in women--Prevention.
  I. Ware, Marsha.   II. Tonnessen, Diana.   III. Title.
  RC931.073N67   1998
  616.7'16--dc21   97-43586
                                                      CIP

Other books by Morris Notelovitz, MD, PhD
    Menopause and Midlife Health (with Diana Tonnessen)
    Estrogen: Yes or No? (with Diana Tonnessen)
    Osteoporosis: Prevention, Diagnosis and Management:
        A Practical Manual for the Primary Care Physician
    The Essential Heart Book for Women (with Diana Tonnessen)

Credits
    Illustrations, pages 14, 18, 20, 21, 27, 32, 34, 76, 87, 90, 121, 122 reprinted from the
        1st edition © 1987 by Triad Communications, Inc.
    Illustrations, pages 16, 31, 71, 72, 73 77 (table), 91 adapted and/or reprinted from
        Osteoporosis: Prevention, Diagnosis and Management © 1994 by Morris Notelovitz.
    Text on pages 117, 154-155, 160–169 from *Osteoporosis: There Is Something You Can
        Do About It!*, © 1997 by Sara Meeks, with the illustrations © 1997 by Gaye Dell

Published and distributed by
    Triad Publishing Company, Post Office Box 13355, Gainesville, FL 32604

To the victims of osteoporosis, including my mother, Fanny Notelovitz. The battle is being won. — M.N.

To my parents, for their gift of education. —M.W.

We wish to thank the staff of the Women's Medical and Diagnostic Center, the Women's Research Center and the Climacteric Clinic, Inc. for their help and cooperation; the numerous volunteers who participated in our studies; our clients for allowing us use of their records; and the women who graciously shared with us and with you their feelings and experiences. It is through their experience that we have been able to develop a preventive and therapeutic program to help you, the reader.

Contents

Foreword

O steoporosis has often been called a "silent disease." This is because it produces absolutely no symptoms until a fracture occurs.

There is, however, another sense in which the disorder is silent, perhaps even invisible. Despite the fact that osteoporosis is an extremely common problem (it is more prevalent than diabetes in postmenopausal women), and despite increased publicity about the disorder in recent years, it is still largely unknown to the general public. A recent survey by the Commonwealth Fund, a national philanthropy, found that seven in ten women are not familiar with it. The authors of *Stand Tall!* attempt to rectify this situation, to overcome the invisibility—the silence—of osteoporosis.

Stand Tall! is a serious effort to provide essential information to the concerned and intelligent layperson. It offers help, but it is not just another self-help book. The authors explain in largely nontechnical language what the scientific community now understands about osteoporosis. The roles of hormones, diet and exercise in causing, preventing and treating this common disorder are discussed and explanations are given of the various tests used.

Osteoporosis research has exploded in the years since *Stand Tall!* was first published in 1982. This new edition does an excellent job of capturing all of this new information.

The book goes a long way toward telling patients with osteoporosis, their families, and those who may develop the disorder both what we know and what we don't know about the problem. It helps to close the gap of unequal knowledge between physician and lay person.

July, 1998

Robert P. Heaney, MD
John A. Creighton University Professor
and Professor of Internal Medicine
Creighton University

Preface

The secret of osteoporosis is out. Most of us now recognize the woman with the dowager's hump as a victim of osteoporosis and not an example of "normal" aging. We are much more aware of good nutrition, exercise and the selective use of hormone therapy than we were a decade ago.

Still, in spite of what we know, more than a million fractures a year continue to be attributed to osteoporosis. Why does the condition continue to threaten the health of so many women? There are several reasons.

Until recently, osteoporosis was viewed as a postmenopausal problem. Thanks to ongoing research, we now recognize that building bone during adolescence and young adulthood is just as important as slowing bone loss after menopause.

Another reason is that most research in the past focused on fractures. Now, scientists have turned their attention to slowing and possibly reversing the invisible loss of bone mass—*osteopenia*—that occurs many years before a fracture. An estimated 20 to 25 million American women have osteopenia and don't know it. Technological improvements now make it possible to accurately test for this invisible loss of bone in its earliest stages, before permanent harm is done.

Scientists recognize that there is no one panacea for preventing osteoporosis premenopausally. Calcium, for example, once touted as the "cure-all," *does* help protect your bones, but is not nearly as effective as calcium with regular moderate exercise. The combination of calcium, exercise and estrogen appears to be the most effective regimen for the majority of menopausal women.

All the advances in prevention, detection and treatment of osteoporosis that have taken place over the sixteen years since the first edition of *Stand Tall* was published are reflected in this new edition.

And we've added more on what you can do in your childbearing years to prevent osteoporosis, more on bone density testing, more on calcium and vitamin D, more on the importance of strong muscles and muscle-strengthening exercises, more on estrogen and progestogen, more on the prevention and treatment of osteoporosis with newer, non-hormonal drugs.

Even good science rarely produces black and white answers, and this is especially true of the research on such a complex medical problem as osteoporosis. Throughout the book, we have tried to guide you through the confusion by making recommendations based on what the majority of studies have shown and on the overall consensus of the medical community. We have also pointed out some of the inconsistencies and unanswered questions in the research because we feel that it is just as important for you to be aware of what is *not* known about osteopososis as what *is* known. Of course, even the advice in this book is subject to change as new and better scientific findings take the place of old ones. So be flexible and try to keep up with the medical advances as much as you can.

While much of the information in this edition has changed, our goal for writing it remains the same. We want to help you understand everything that is currently known about osteoporosis and how it can affect your health, so you can make educated decisions about your own life and take a stand against osteoporosis now.

Morris Notelovitz
Marsha Ware
Diana Tonnessen

Stand Tall!

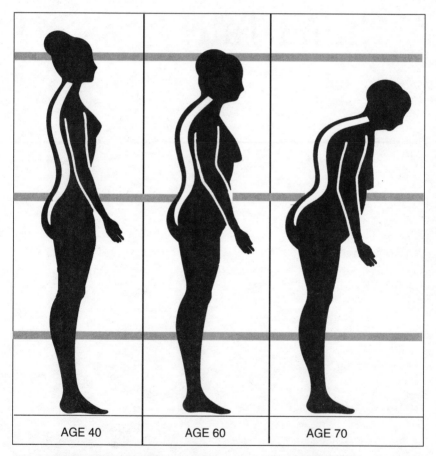

AGE 40	AGE 60	AGE 70

THE SHRINKING WOMAN. When spinal vertebrae weakened by osteoporosis collapse, it causes loss of height (all from the upper part of the body), inward curvature
of the lower spine, outward curvature of the upper spine, and protruding of the
abdomen.

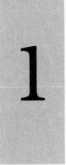

1 Understanding the Problem

More than half of all women will experience osteoporotic fractures during their lives. The process of losing bone is painless and takes place gradually, over many years. The frightening reality is that you can't see when your bones get thin, and there are no warning symptoms prior to a fracture.

Scientists divide this loss of bone into two separate conditions: *osteopenia* and *osteoporosis*. The difference between them is a matter of degree.

OSTEOPENIA

A certain amount of age-related bone loss is normal and, as far as we know, inevitable. Age-related changes result in a decrease in the spongy (trabecular) bone that is characteristic of the spine. But if loss of bone occurs at a faster pace than that associated with normal aging, and if it progresses to the point that about 10 to 25%

of bone mass is lost from the amount of bone you had in your mid-30s (based on an estimate of average peak bone mass in a group of "young normal" women), the condition that results is called *osteopenia.* If nothing is done to slow or stop bone loss, the process may continue until it turns into actual osteoporosis. Eventually, bones may fracture.

Osteopenia is a risk factor for osteoporosis just as high blood pressure is a risk factor for heart disease and stroke. And, just

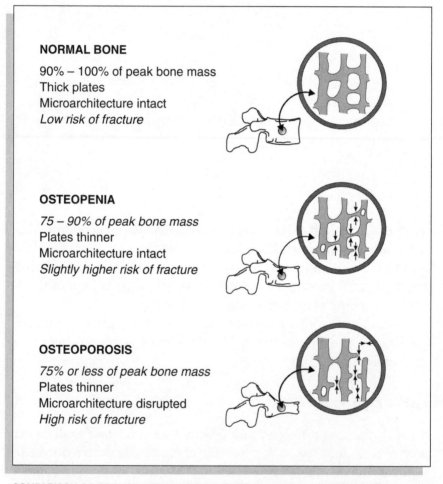

NORMAL BONE

90% – 100% of peak bone mass
Thick plates
Microarchitecture intact
Low risk of fracture

OSTEOPENIA

75 – 90% of peak bone mass
Plates thinner
Microarchitecture intact
Slightly higher risk of fracture

OSTEOPOROSIS

75% or less of peak bone mass
Plates thinner
Microarchitecture disrupted
High risk of fracture

COMPARISON OF NORMAL AND ABNORMAL BONE IN A SPINAL VERTEBRA. *Top:* normal bone. *Center: osteopenia.* Decrease in the spongy (trabecular) bone that is characteristic of the spine. *Bottom: osteoporosis.* Erosion and perforations have developed in the delicate plates that make up the bone's honeycomb structure.

as with high blood pressure, there are no symptoms. You could lose bone mass for years without realizing it.

The earlier osteopenia is detected, the more likely you will be able to reduce your risk of developing osteoporosis.

Osteopenia is a risk factor for osteoporosis.

OSTEOPOROSIS

Osteoporosis (Latin for *porous bone*) is a reduction in bone mass to the point that the bones become fragile—weak enough to easily lead to a broken hip, crushed vertebra or fractured wrist. Osteoporotic bone is no different from normal bone; there is just less of it.

In the early stages, there may be microscopic fractures that you are not aware of. Later, when the bones are no longer strong enough to withstand the physical stresses of everyday activity, more serious fractures can result; sometimes there is no apparent cause. The causes and mechanisms of osteoporosis are complex and varied, but the end result is always the same: porous, weak, fragile bones that are easily broken.

Osteoporotic bone does not differ from normal bone; there is just less of it.

There are two types of bone in the skeleton, and osteoporosis may be classified by which type is more severely affected as well as how rapidly bone is lost.

- *Postmenopausal osteoporosis* is most common just after menopause. It affects the meshlike trabecular bone primarily (as in the spine) and is characterized by a rapid loss of bone.

- *Aging* or *senile osteoporosis* usually occurs after age 70. It affects both trabecular and cortical bone (the compact bone that constitutes much of the tubular framework of the long bones) and is characterized by a slower rate of bone loss. It is thought to be an exaggeration of the bone loss that occurs normally with age.

Both of these are called "primary" osteoporosis. When osteoporosis results from a specific cause, such as a chronic medical condition or the use of certain drugs, it is called "secondary."

WHICH BONES BREAK
WHEN YOU HAVE OSTEOPOROSIS?

Fractures of the spinal vertebrae, the wrist and the hip are most commonly associated with osteoporosis, although broken bones in other parts of the skeleton are not unusual. Having even one fracture is a sign of a weakened skeleton, and your risk of another fracture is greatly increased. Other fractures can be in the same

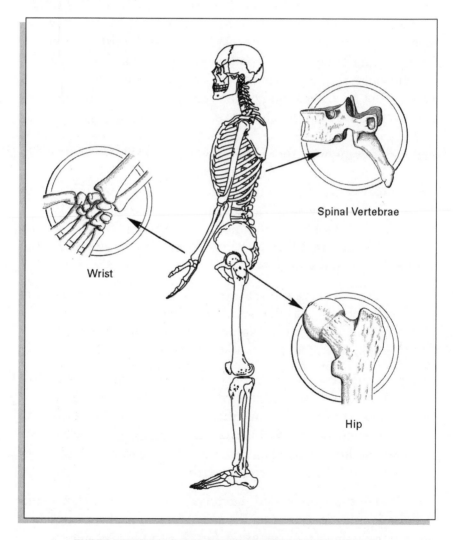

Spinal Vertebrae

Wrist

Hip

THREE PRINCIPAL SITES OF OSTEOPOROTIC FRACTURES

or a different part of the body. Osteoporosis is a so-called "hetero-geneous" condition, which means you can have normal bone mass in the spine and osteoporosis in the hip, or vice versa.

Spinal vertebrae   Because the bones of the spine are com-posed primarily of the meshlike trabecular bone, they are usually the first to show the effects of osteoporosis. As the years of losing bone take their toll and the vertebrae become more porous and weak, they go through various stages of structural deformity. In time, they can actually collapse.

Vertebral fractures are most likely to occur between the ages of 50 and 70. Up to one-third of all women over age 60, and half of all white women over age 85, have one or more vertebral fractures.

These fractures usually follow a sudden attempt to straighten the spine from a flexed (forward bending) posi-tion. This is a common movement that is part of such everyday activities as opening a window, lifting groceries or making a bed.

A fracture can result from something as ordinary as making a bed.

Fractures can also occur spontaneously as weakened bones simply give way under the weight of the body.

Stages of spinal collapse. In the first stages of bone collapse, the affected vertebra takes on a biconcave shape (curved inward at the top and bottom) in a vain attempt to maintain the structural in-tegrity of the spine and support the weight of the body. When two adjacent vertebrae are affected, the space between them becomes fish-shaped; the word *"codfishing"* is used to describe this.

Eventually the strain is too much, and the anterior (front) side of the bone collapses, producing the characteristic *wedge fracture*. As the process continues, the posterior (back) side may collapse as well, resulting in a totally collapsed vertebra. This is called a *crush fracture*. Wedge and crush fractures occur most often in the region of the upper lumbar vertebrae (middle of the back) and mid to lower thoracic, because these parts of the spine bear most of the weight.

Symptoms of spinal fracture. About half the women who have had a spinal fracture do not recall having had back pain. Their fractures are sometimes detected with a routine x-ray. But other women have severe pain, sometimes with permanent lower back pain. When

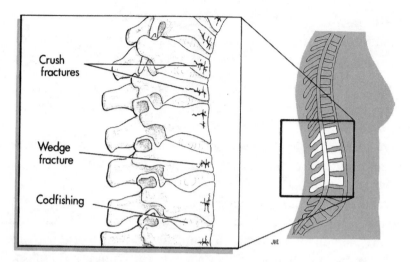

STAGES OF VERTEBRAL COLLAPSE. 1. *Codfishing:* affected vertebrae curve inward at top and bottom in an attempt to support the weight of the body; term describes the fish-shaped space that results when two adjacent vertebrae are affected. 2. *Wedge fracture:* anterior (front) side of the bone collapses. 3. C*rush fracture:* produced when the posterior (back) side collapses as well, resulting in a totally collapsed vertebra.

there is pain, it typically follows the same pattern.

First there is an *acute phase,* with intense pain localized at the site of the fracture. This pain is due not only to the fracture itself, but also to damage to the surrounding tissues. There may also be muscle spasm and pain down the legs. This stage usually lasts from four to eight weeks, until the bone heals in the new collapsed form.

The *chronic phase* then follows, and it can last from six months to a year. The pain during this period is a less severe "burning" or "tired" feeling, largely due to muscle spasm and ligament strain. The change in posture resulting from the spinal deformity—usually a forward rotation of the shoulders—also creates muscle tension and pain. Though the intensity may ease, if the spinal deformity presses on nerves some pain nearly always remains.

After the chronic phase has passed, a woman is said to be in *remission,* and she may have no pain or muscle spasms . . . until she fractures another vertebra.

How the body is affected. If several vertebrae collapse, as is

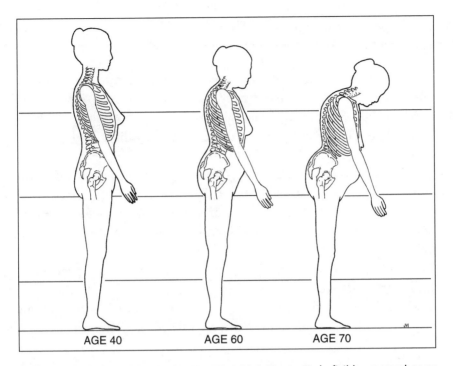

AGE 40   AGE 60   AGE 70

EFFECTS OF SPINAL COLLAPSE (The "Shrinking Woman"). *Left:* this woman has no outward signs of osteoporosis. Without a bone density test, she cannot know if her bones are getting so fragile they will fracture later. *Center:* some spinal fractures result in early signs of osteoporosis. *Right:* if fracturing continues, there can be significant loss of height, tilted rib cage, dowager's hump, inward curvature of the lower spine and a protruding abdomen.

often the case, five may fill the space normally occupied by three. Continued fractures can cause the rib cage to tilt downward toward the hips, eventually coming to rest on the hip bones. The outcome is outward curvature of the upper spine (*kyphosis*), leading to a dowager's hump, inward curvature of the lower spine (*lordosis*), and a protruding abdomen because the downward movement of the ribs forces the internal organs outward. The spine may hunch, squeezing internal organs and impairing breathing and digestion.

Height loss usually occurs in bursts of one-half to one inch or more, corresponding to the number of vertebrae that have collapsed. It is not unusual for a woman with osteoporosis to become as much as two inches shorter in just a few weeks. Eventually, she may lose a total of eight inches or more from her adult height, all from the upper part of her body. There is no change in the length of the long bones of the arms and legs.

The wrist   It's natural to extend your arm to break a fall. But when you do, the result may be a wrist fracture (sometimes called a *Colles' fracture)*. Although broken wrist bones usually heal easily and do not lead to any subsequent disability, they serve as a warning of cortical bone loss.

The lower part of the *radius* (the shorter and thicker of the two forearm bones) contains about 25% trabecular and 75% cortical bone. Loss of both types results in a thinning and weakening of the radius and accounts for the sharp rise in wrist fractures in women over the age of 50.

Later, as women get older, they get fewer fractures of the wrist and more fractures of the hip. The reason has to do with how people fall. Younger women fall forward and extend their arm to break the fall. Older women tend to fall backward, which increases the risk of landing on their hip.

The hip   Hip fractures—more accurately, fractures of the upper part of the femur (the thigh bone)—are without a doubt the most disabling and life-threatening consequence of osteoporosis. If you are a 50-year-old white woman, your risk of having a hip fracture at some point in your life is estimated to be 17%—equivalent to your *combined* risk of breast, uterine and ovarian cancer. Black women have a much lower incidence of hip fractures than white women.

Long ago it was thought that women were more susceptible to hip fractures than men were because they tripped over their long skirts. We now know that women break their hips more often because they have lost more bone. The fracture is frequently from trauma that healthy bones could easily withstand, but sometimes there is no apparent cause at all. That leads to the unanswerable question: did she break her hip because she fell, or did she fall because she broke her hip?

Because of the relatively larger proportion of cortical bone in the upper femur, and because she is more likely to fall backward, it is the older woman with advanced osteoporosis who is most likely to fracture her hip. Those who survive are likely to fracture the other hip.

Medical treatment and consequences. A hip fracture requires immediate medical attention. Metal pins or screws are used to join the broken sections of the bone. Severe fractures may require replacement of the femoral head with a prosthetic (artificial) device. The patient is usually hospitalized for five to seven days. Recovery depends on the severity of the fracture and the age and general health of the patient.

About half of all women who suffer a hip fracture die within the first year following the injury. Death is not caused by the fracture itself but by some condition arising from confinement to a hospital or nursing home bed, such as pneumonia, thrombosis (blood clots) or a fat embolism (fat that enters the bloodstream and becomes trapped in the lung). Of the women who survive, half will never regain the quality of life they had before, and 15 to 25% of those who were living independently before the injury can no longer do so, but remain in long-term health care institutions.

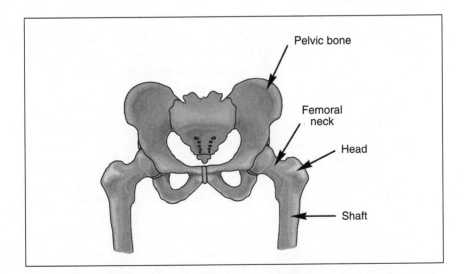

WHAT BONES BREAK WHEN A HIP FRACTURES? A hip fracture is actually a fracture of the upper part of the thigh bone (the femur). Most fractures occur at the neck, which is the weakest part, although the shaft or head of the femur can also break.

Case report: Eve, age 67   Eve was an attractive, healthy woman crippled "overnight" by physical deformity and paralyzing pain. Her life was prematurely shortened by a trivial accident that would normally result in nothing more than a slight bruise and a sore leg.

Eve was 67 when she experienced the first of a series of vertebral fractures. As the fracturing continued, her height dropped from 5'7" to 4'11", and she was in a great deal of pain. Spinal x-rays showed two wedge fractures and eight crush fractures.

She described how osteoporosis affected her life and her attitudes about herself and those around her . . .

The first fracture happened when my husband and I were moving some furniture around the house. Because I was always strong and never hesitated to move things, I picked up a chair to take it into the garage. As I opened the door and put down the chair I heard something crack in my back. It was painful, but I thought I was all right. We even went to a party that night, although a friend told me she could see the pain in my face.

The pain got progressively worse over the next couple of months. Any movement of my back, chest or ribs was absolute agony—the pain was excruciating. I had trouble sleeping because even lying down hurt so badly. By this time I was nearly crippled. I couldn't bend or stoop. The pain would be so bad I'd cry sometimes.

After a while the pain started to subside and I could get around a little. My husband would ask me to come outside with him for a bit and that would make me feel better.

Eventually I could go out shopping for a short time. I didn't really want to go anywhere, though. People who knew me didn't recognize me. I didn't want to see anybody because of the way I looked.

One of the hardest things is finding clothes. I can't get into anything anymore. I can't dress and look like anybody because of the hump on my back. By the time I get something to fit around the hump and around my stomach, it's too big everywhere else. My legs are still long but I'm so short and wide on top. It's hard because I used to love clothes. My husband won't go shopping with me anymore because it hurts him so much to see me try to get into clothes.

A problem that most people wouldn't think of is going to a restaurant. The tables are too high. I feel like a little kid who needs a booster seat. I can practically push the food off my plate into my mouth. Now I take cushions with me to sit on and it's much better.

Sometimes I get very self-conscious and feel like everyone is looking at me. I don't like to be with people we used to know because they look at me and wonder what happened. I'd rather meet new people who can't compare me to what I used to look like.

I know now that what I have is osteoporosis and that it took years for it to develop. But I didn't know then. It would be good for young women to find out about osteoporosis and for their doctors to be conscientious and tell them what they can do to prevent it.

Eve's story illustrates how the pain, deformity and disability that resulted from osteoporosis profoundly affected her emotional well-being. She knew she would never again look the way she used to. Her independence suffered, as she had to rely on family and friends to fulfill the simplest of needs.

Eighteen months after giving this interview, Eve's husband called her to look at the kitchen floor he had just cleaned. When Eve stepped onto the wet floor, she slipped and broke her hip. Six days later she died, following complications after "successful" surgery.

* * *

With our better understanding of how bone is formed and the technology that allows accurate and precise measuring of a woman's bone mass and her rate of bone loss, osteoporosis has become a preventable condition. The key is to build bone mass when you're young and to regulate the rate at which it is lost after menopause. How this may be achieved is discussed in the following chapters.

2 Your Bones and How They Change

Your skeleton consists of 206 bones, and they are truly remarkable! Though they are among the hardest tissues in the body, they are flexible enough to enable you to run, jump, bend and twist.

That is, if you take care of them. How you take care of your bones will determine how long they will last and how well they will do the job they were meant to do.

- Bones offer support and protection to the body.

- Bones enable you to move around.

- Bones manufacture blood cells and store 99% of your body's calcium.

You may be surprised to learn that bones are not solid, as they appear, but are living tissues richly supplied with blood vessels, nerve fibers and fluid-filled channels. Bones are actually among the most complex tissues in your body. Throughout your life, they will be influenced by your heredity, hormones, diet, physical activity, stress, injury, disease and drugs. It is not an exaggeration to say that almost everything that happens to you also has an effect on your bones.

An inside look Every bone in your skeleton is made up of two kinds of bone. Each has a different structural makeup:

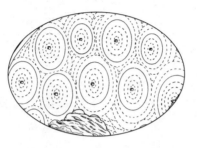

Cortical bone looks solid and dense, with a circular pattern resembling the whorls in cut wood.

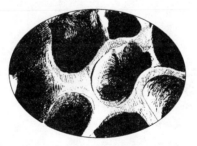

Trabecular bone is porous and looks like a honeycomb.

In every bone, the trabecular bone is surrounded by cortical bone. But their proportions differ—from one bone to another and even within parts of an individual bone. The vertebrae of your spine, for example, consist mostly of porous trabecular bone surrounded by a thin cortical shell. At the other extreme are the hard, long bones of your arms and legs, which are mostly cortical with areas of trabecular bone at both ends.

Trabecular bone, despite its delicate appearance, is actually very

HOW NEW BONE IS MADE
THE REMODELING CYCLE OF TRABECULAR BONE

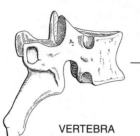

VERTEBRA

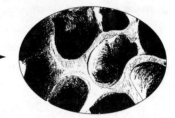

TRABECULAR PLATE of a
vertebra (magnified 1,000 times)

1. **BREAKDOWN:** The cycle begins on the surface of each trabecular plate
   with activation of dormant cells, called *osteoclast precursors*, into bone-
   breakdown cells called *osteoclasts*.

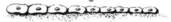

   The *osteoclasts* release an acid-like substance that dissolves old bone
   and digs microscopic cavities along the surfaces of the bone.

2. **BONE FORMATION:** Bone forming cells, called *osteoblasts*, are attracted to
   the cavities made by the osteoclasts. There, they begin producing a soft
   collagen matrix to fill the cavities.

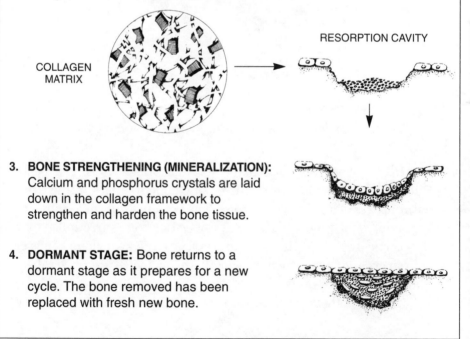

COLLAGEN
MATRIX

RESORPTION CAVITY

3. **BONE STRENGTHENING (MINERALIZATION):**
   Calcium and phosphorus crystals are laid
   down in the collagen framework to
   strengthen and harden the bone tissue.

4. **DORMANT STAGE:** Bone returns to a
   dormant stage as it prepares for a new
   cycle. The bone removed has been
   replaced with fresh new bone.

strong; its latticework structure of vertical and horizontal plates provides maximum support with a minimum of material. But all those fine surfaces create an enormous amount of exposed area, and so more bone loss can occur there.

HOW NEW BONE IS MADE

Like all living tissue, bone is constantly being broken down and re-formed. This cyclic process takes place on the surface of each bone. It is called *bone remodeling.* (In young people whose bones are growing and changing shape, the process is called bone *modeling.*)

Bone remodeling takes place continuously throughout your life, as old, weak or damaged bone tissue is replaced with new bone. The cycle lasts about 3 to 4 months.

Each cycle consists of four parts:

1. Bone breakdown   The cycle begins with the activation of dormant cells *(osteoclast precursors),* which turn into breakdown cells called *osteoclasts.* The osteoclasts release an acid-like substance that dissolves old bone and digs microscopic cavities along the surfaces of the bone.

2. Bone formation   Bone forming cells, called *osteoblasts,* are attracted to the cavities made by the osteoclasts. The osteoblasts start producing a soft collagen matrix to fill the cavities.

3. Bone strengthening   Calcium and phosphorus crystals are laid down into this collagen framework, to strengthen and harden the bone tissue, in a process called *bone mineralization.* Mature osteoblasts, called *osteocytes,* are embedded in the hardened bone; osteocytes are believed to play a role in storage of calcium and repair of microfractures.

4. Dormant stage   Once the old bone has been replaced with an equivalent amount of new bone, the cells again become dormant, as they prepare for a new cycle.

WHAT ARE BONES MADE OF?

Bone tissue is composed of tiny crystals of calcium and phosphorus embedded in a framework of interlocking protein fibers (primarily collagen).

The calcium crystals give your bones their strength, hardness and rigidity. The collagen fibers give them their relative "shock absorbing" capacity for flexibility, which allows bone to bend a little instead of breaking under stress.

A number of other materials are also present in bone: fluoride, sodium, potassium, magnesium and citrate, plus a host of trace elements. These act as the "mortar" holding the "bricks" of calcium and phosphorus crystals together.

HOW DO BONES GET FRAGILE?

Your *bone mass*—the total amount of bone in your skeleton—is controlled by the bone remodeling cycle. The cycle maintains a delicate balance of bone breakdown and new bone formation that changes constantly in response to the needs of your body. (By some estimates, 10% of cortical bone and 30 to 40% of trabecular bone is remodeled each year.)

The loss of bone mass begins when the remodeling process "uncouples," and there is more bone breakdown than new bone formation. The normal balance between breakdown and formation is replaced by a different pattern: either formation of new bone is slowed, or breakdown becomes faster.

- *Decreased bone formation*: the activity of the bone-breakdown osteoclasts remains normal, but that of the bone-building osteoblasts is slowed. Women with this pattern of bone loss are sometimes called "slow losers."

- *Rapid bone breakdown*: new bone formation by osteoblasts is normal, but bone breakdown is faster than normal. The result—rapid and excessive losses of bone mass—is characteristic of the years immediately following menopause. Women with this pattern of bone loss are sometimes called "fast losers."

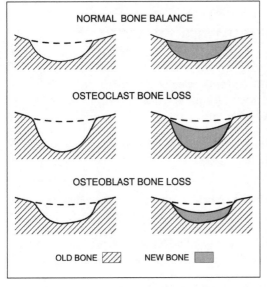

HOW BONE IS LOST

Normal bone balance: *Left:* resorption cavity of normal depth. *Right:* cavity completely refilled with new bone.

Osteoclast bone loss: *Left:* resorption cavity of excessive depth. *Right:* cavity only partly refilled by a normal amount of new bone.

Osteoblast bone loss: *Left:* resorption cavity of normal depth. *Right:* cavity only partly refilled by a subnormal amount of new bone.

If nothing is done to prevent it, excessive bone tissue can be lost. Once that happens, the bones become vulnerable to structural damage. The porous trabecular bone is most vulnerable. So, if there are imbalances in the remodeling process, the spinal vertebrae are likely to be affected first. Osteoclasts can cause so much erosion that perforations form in the delicate plates that make up the honeycomb structure—in effect, weakening or breaking some of the pillar supports of the bone.

Later, as the destructive process continues, cortical bone is affected as well, and it starts getting thinner.

HOW YOUR AGE AFFECTS YOUR BONES

Your skeleton, just as the rest of your body, changes as it gets older. In the early years, the changes are very visible; later changes are less obvious.

Childhood From birth until early adulthood, your body produces more bone tissue than it loses through bone breakdown. A child's skeleton enlarges because the amount of new tissue formed

HOW BONE CHANGES WITH AGE

All bone has three surfaces, called *envelopes:* the *periosteal envelope* (the outer surface), the *endosteal envelope* (the inner surface, facing the marrow cavity), and the *intracortical envelope* (the material in between). All three have identical cell makeup.

Throughout childhood, new bone formation takes place on the outer (periosteal) envelope and a lesser amount of breakdown occurs on the inner (endosteal) envelope.

During adolescence, bone forms on both surfaces, leading to large over-all gains in bone mass.

During early adulthood, breakdown begins again on the inner (endosteal) envelope—the beginning of the age-related decline in bone mass.

(Bone loss associated with immobilization or prolonged bed rest takes place in the intracortical envelope.)

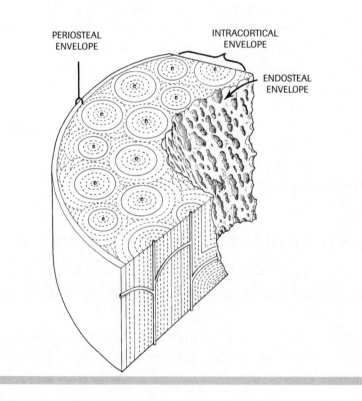

on the outer surfaces of the bones exceeds the amount broken down on the inner surfaces.

Adolescence   The teen years bring about an acceleration in growth that is related to the surge in sex hormone production. Estrogen and progesterone in girls, and androgens in boys, stimulate formation of new bone on the outer surfaces. Later, more bone is added on the inner surfaces and in the intracortical envelopes. The growth spurts that adolescents have are due to the laying down of new bone tissue on both inner and outer surfaces of existing bone.

Adulthood   Although it eventually slows somewhat, this pattern of growth continues into adulthood. Then the childhood pattern of bone remodeling resumes, with outer surface formation and inner surface breakdown. Now, however, the rate of breakdown exceeds that of new formation, and bone mass begins to decline.

HOW YOUR SEX AFFECTS YOUR BONES

Both women and men lose bone as they get older; the difference is in the rate of that loss. At skeletal maturity, men generally have bigger bones and more bone mass than women, and so they can withstand age-related losses of bone mass better than women.

In addition, the two types of bone tissue follow different patterns of bone loss in men and women:

Trabecular bone. Unbelievable as it seems, many authorities believe that decline of bone mass begins—for both sexes—in the mid-twenties, with the loss of trabecular bone from the spine. Most research suggests that women lose 1.2% of trabecular bone each year, beginning about ten years before menopause and continuing throughout the rest of their lives. Other studies indicate that both men and women lose small but significant amounts of trabecular bone in the spine before age 50.

Bone mass begins to decline in the mid-20s.

Women, however, have a dramatically accelerated rate of bone loss after menopause. Some women lose as much as 50% of their spinal bone density during the first ten years after menopause.

Cortical bone. In both sexes, cortical bone mass reaches its peak around age 30 to 35, followed by a slight loss (between .3% to .5% per year) until about 50; this loss comes primarily from the long bones of the arms and legs. But then a woman, if she has undergone menopause, will begin losing cortical bone at a rate of 2% to 3% per year—*up to six times faster than a man does.*

Women lose bone most rapidly in the first 5 to 6 years following menopause; the pattern of bone loss is

By age 55, a woman may lose the same amount of bone she gained during her adolescent growth phase. the mirror image of the growth spurt that followed adolescent hormone surges. If she does nothing to prevent it, it is estimated that by the time she reaches the age of 55, the bone lost may be equivalent to that gained during her adolescent growth phase.

Around age 65, her rate of bone loss begins to slow down, again becoming similar to that of men. (But even though the rate of loss slows, she has already lost a great deal more bone than a man.) Both women and men then continue to slowly, but steadily, lose bone as a natural part of the aging process.

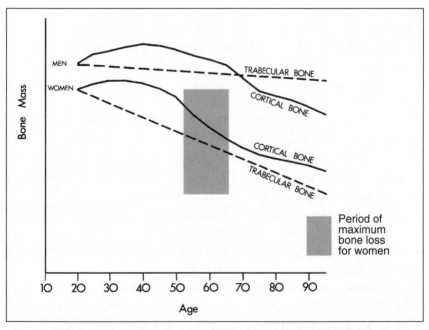

BONE LOSS WITH AGE: A COMPARISON OF MEN AND WOMEN

3 How Your Body Regulates Bone Mass

Throughout your life, your bones are regulated by numerous complex interactions involving calcium, phosphorus, vitamin D, estrogen and a number of other hormones. The bones themselves also produce powerful substances that help regulate bone mass.

Calcium and phosphorus are the most abundant substances in the human body. Both are intimately involved in the regulation of metabolism, including bone metabolism. There are literally thousands of chemical reactions in the body that sense and respond to changes in calcium and phosphorus.

If any of these stops functioning properly, your skeleton can start losing bone.

Note: The subject of this chapter may be difficult to absorb with the first reading. It is included so you can see the complexities of how bone loss occurs, and to provide insights into the ways scientists look for ways to prevent bone loss. We have tried to explain it in understandable terms.

CALCIUM AND THE "BONE HORMONES"

In addition to calcium's important role in bone physiology (99% of your body's calcium is in your skeleton), it

Your body will sacrifice bone mass to keep enough calcium in your blood.

is essential for normal muscle contraction, heart function, blood clotting and regulation of blood pressure.

Because calcium is so vital, the human body has evolved an elaborate system of hormonal checks and balances—a sort of "calcium thermostat"—to ensure there is always enough of it in your bloodstream.

Estrogen For many years, scientists have been aware of a close association between the beginning of the body's loss of estrogen at menopause and accelerated bone loss. It appears to make

Loss of estrogen leads to loss of bone.

no difference whether the menopause is natural or surgical: a 45-year-old woman whose ovaries were removed at age 35 will have as little bone mass as a 60-year-old woman who had a natural menopause at 50 (unless she takes estrogen).

In contrast, women whose bodies still manufacture estrogen so they are still menstruating in their 50s typically have normal or only slightly reduced bone mass until they stop menstruating. Then they begin the typical pattern of postmenopausal bone loss.

Bone loss at menopause. Bone loss is most pronounced in the first 5 or 6 years after menopause and finally slows down at around age 65. At the same time, there is a dramatic decline in production

Bone loss is most severe in the first 5 or 6 years after menopause.

of the female sex hormones, estrogen and progesterone, by the ovaries. The bone loss that follows menopause is a consequence of the body's loss of these two hormones.

Younger women with low estrogen levels may experience the same pattern of bone loss. It would therefore seem that these hormones protect the bones in some way and that when their levels drop, the protection is lost.

The estrogen-bone connection. Various tissues in the body have receptors to attract estrogen, and estrogen has a direct effect on these tissues. The breasts and lining of the uterus have estrogen receptors. Trabecular bone cells have almost as many estrogen receptors as the uterine lining. This is why estrogen has a direct, protective effect on bone.

In addition, estrogen interacts with the other hormones to preserve bone mass. It is believed that estrogen affects bone directly in the following ways:

- Increases the number and activity of the bone-building cells (osteoblasts), and reduces the activity of the bone-removing cells (osteoclasts);

- Increases collagen production by osteoblasts;

- Increases activity of certain growth factors in bone, notably transforming growth factor beta;

- Stimulates progesterone receptors in bone (progesterone appears to have its own protective effects on bone).

Progesterone   Bone tissue has, in addition to estrogen receptors, progesterone receptors that are stimulated by estrogen. Progesterone is the female hormone produced by the ovaries during the second half of the menstrual cycle. It is thought to help protect bone mass by increasing the activity of bone-building osteoblasts, and by preventing the adrenal hormones from breaking down bone tissue:

> Jerilyn C. Prior, MD, found that menstruating women with normal blood levels of estrogen but low levels of progesterone lost up to 4% of their bone mass over a one-year period, but women with higher progesterone levels did not lose bone mass.

> In a 10-year study, Lila Nachtigall, MD, found that women who started taking estrogen and a progestogen (synthetic form of progesterone) within three years after menopause showed an increase in bone density. Women who started therapy more than three years after menopause had some loss of bone density, but not as much as the women who took no hormones at all.

A study by Claus Christiansen, MD, showed that bone density increased during the three years that postmenopausal women took a combination of estrogen and progestogen.

Androgens Although we typically think of androgens (testosterone and related hormones) as "male" reproductive hormones, small amounts are produced by the ovaries and adrenal glands in women. Testosterone is thought to protect bone by directly stimulating osteoblasts and enhancing the body's production of the hormone *calcitonin*. Evidence is mounting that androgens play a role in maintaining bone health:

In a two-year study of surgically menopausal women we conducted in conjunction with researchers at Duke and Emory universities, those on estrogen alone had less than a 1% increase in spinal bone density, while those on an estrogen-testosterone combination had a 3.4% increase. The biggest gains in density (6.5%) were in women taking the combination who had not had estrogen for at least two years before entering the study.

Most transsexual men who are treated with drugs that suppress the body's production of androgen have decreased bone formation and some even begin to lose bone mass. This happens even though they are also taking estrogen.

Vitamin D Vitamin D is probably more correctly considered a hormone than a vitamin. It comes from the sun (produced by the ultraviolet irradiation of an inactive form of vitamin D in your skin) and in limited amounts from foods such as eggs, milk and fish. Like *parathyroid hormone*, vitamin D helps maintain a proper level of calcium in the blood.

The right amount of vitamin D is beneficial. But too much can cause bone loss.

The correct amount of vitamin D is beneficial: it helps to maintain a positive calcium balance and it is even used to treat women with osteoporosis. But an excess can have the reverse effect and *actually withdraw calcium from the bones, leading to bone loss.*

A high level of estrogen in the body, such as during pregnancy, stimulates the activation of vitamin D. But it is not known if a drop in estrogen, as occurs at menopause, prevents vitamin D to be activated.

This is what we do know:

- Postmenopausal women who have osteoporosis are less able than other postmenopausal women to complete the last step of vitamin D activation in the kidney.

- Both oral contraceptives and postmenopausal hormone therapy enhance the activation of vitamin D.

Parathyroid hormone   The parathyroids are four tiny glands in your neck. If the calcium in your blood should fall too low (remember, calcium is vital for normal muscle contraction, heart function and other processes in the body), these glands release parathyroid hormone into the bloodstream to increase the level of calcium. As a result:

Parathyroid hormone keeps enough calcium in the blood by taking it from the bones.

- The kidneys put calcium back into the bloodstream (this calcium would otherwise be excreted in the urine).

- Vitamin D is converted to an active form, which allows the intestines to absorb more calcium from your food.

- *Bone is broken down,* to release stored calcium into the bloodstream.

Estrogen normally reduces this bone-dissolving action. But when estrogen levels fall after menopause, even a small amount of parathyroid hormone stimulates bone loss. To make matters worse, the calcium released from the broken-down bone raises the level of calcium in the bloodstream, which turns off the calcium "thermostat" in the parathyroid gland. Then the kidneys begin to secrete calcium in the urine, setting the stage for even more bone loss.

Calcitonin   This hormone, released mainly by the thyroid gland, protects bones from the dissolving effects of parathyroid hormone and excessive vitamin D. Because of these actions it is often referred to as a "calcium-sparing" hormone.

How it works is not completely understood, but there is evidence to suggest that calcitonin inhibits the activity of the cells that break down bone (osteoclasts). We know this:

- Men have more calcitonin than women;

- Women with osteoporosis have less calcitonin than those with a normal amount of bone;

- African-American women have more calcitonin than white women (which may help explain why they are less predisposed to develop osteoporosis);

- Calcitonin decreases with age (which may be another reason we all lose bone as we get older);

- Calcitonin increases with estrogen, both during pregnancy and with estrogen therapy after menopause;

- Calcitonin declines in surgically menopausal women. (But there haven't been enough studies to know if the loss of estrogen after a natural menopause leads to a decline in calcitonin.)

Adrenal hormones   Overactivity of the adrenal gland is frequently associated with severe osteoporosis. The same is true for long-term use of drugs that resemble adrenal hormones, such as cortisone.

A number of adrenal hormones, known collectively as *glucocorticoids,* act directly on bone. They attach to receptors on the surface of bone cells (much like metal objects attach to a magnet) and cause the bone to become more susceptible to the dissolving effects of parathyroid hormone and excessive amounts of vitamin D.

Estrogen stimulates the liver to produce a protein that binds to some of the adrenal hormones, lessening their ability to dissolve bone. This effect stops with the loss of estrogen during the years just after menopause. Sometime after the 65th year, the production of adrenal hormones slows down. Some scientists refer to this as the "adrenopause" and think it is the reason that the rate of bone loss decreases at this time.

Growth hormone   As its name implies, this hormone (secreted mainly from the pituitary gland) stimulates growth of many tissues, one of which is bone. Dwarfs have a deficiency of growth hormone; giants have an excess of it.

In bone tissue, the bone-building cells (osteoblasts) contain receptors for growth hormone, which helps stimulate the production of more osteoblasts without increasing the bone-breakdown activity of osteoclasts. As a result, new bone is formed faster than old bone is broken down, resulting in an overall increase in bone mass.

The production of growth hormone is higher in premenopausal women than in postmenopausal women. *The differences are linked to estrogen; the higher the level of estrogen, the higher the level of growth hormone.*

Thyroid hormone   This hormone plays an important role in the early development of the skeleton. A deficiency in children leads to stunted growth, and an excess in either children or adults leads to an increase in the rate of bone breakdown, resulting in bone loss.

Estrogen stimulates the liver to produce proteins that bind thyroid hormone (in a manner similar to the adrenal hormones), which reduces its ability to break down bone. After menopause, there is less such binding. But we don't know whether or not the increased amount of unbound or "free" thyroid hormone after menopause is important in terms of bone loss.

HOW THE BONES HELP REGULATE THEIR OWN BONE MASS

The bones themselves regulate the bone remodeling cycle via *electrical impulses, prostaglandins* and *growth factors.*

Electrical impulses   Certain tissues in the body generate electrical currents that stimulate and control your heartbeat and other bodily functions. Bone, too, is capable of creating electrical impulses, and these somehow stimulate the formation of new bone.

Since the early 1970s, low-energy electrical currents have been used successfully to treat broken bones that wouldn't heal. *It is possible that electrical current created when bones are physically stressed—as when you exercise—is the reason why exercise builds bone mass.*

Prostaglandins   These substances are produced in many tissues throughout the body: bone, brain, breasts, blood vessels, gastrointestinal tract, kidneys and reproductive tract. They are believed to play an important role in the regulation of many different bodily functions, including bone formation. Some researchers believe that prostaglandins may help osteoclasts and osteoblasts communicate with each other—for instance, helping the bone-breakdown osteoclasts prompt the bone-building osteoblasts into action.

Growth factors   Growth factors are responsible for tissue repair and regeneration throughout the body. Some growth factors, such as *insulin-like growth factor* (IGF), have been found to stimulate bone formation; others actually inhibit it.

A growth factor produced by osteoblasts—perhaps one of the most important—is called *transforming growth factor beta* (TGF-beta). It is known to stimulate growth in other tissues in the body and *it is believed to stimulate the formation of new bone.* Researchers hope that TGF-beta may one day be useful as a therapy in the prevention and treatment of osteopososis.

4 Assessing Your Risk

A re you at risk for osteoporosis? If you knew, you could start taking steps to stop it from happening. Or if you knew you were not at risk you could safely ignore the problem.

A variety of clues are available to help you assess your personal risk. Based on studies of large groups of women, researchers have discovered what makes some women more likely to develop osteoporosis than others. The more of these *risk factors* you have, the more likely you are to lose bone mass.

Even the best research, however, does not provide hard and fast answers. Results sometimes differ from one study to another. In some cases a risk factor for one woman can actually be protective for another.

This chapter will help you evaluate your own risk for osteoporosis and, where possible, suggest what you can do about it.

HEREDITY

Osteoporosis results from a complex interplay of many factors, of which heredity is one of the most influential. Genes play an important role in determining how much bone you have at maturity and your subequent rate of bone loss. Some day we may be able to identify those genes. For the present, however, turn to your family history. If your mother, sister, grandmother or aunt has osteoporosis, you are at higher risk. How do we know?

If someone in your family has osteoporosis, your own risk is higher.

- Many, if not most, women with osteoporosis have a family history of the disorder.

- Identical twins, who have identical genes, have more closely matched bone mass than fraternal twins.

- In an Australian study, premenopausal women whose mothers had osteoporosis had spinal bone density averaging 7% lower than women of the same age who had no family history. In the hip it was 5% lower.

What you can do. If you have a family history of osteoporosis or other hereditary risk factors, you can reduce your risk by eating properly, getting enough calcium, exercising regularly and, when menopause approaches, asking your doctor if you are a candidate for hormone therapy or for one of the other bone conserving drugs. A bone density test is the only way to know for sure if you have low bone mass.

A bone density test is the only way to know for sure if you have low bone mass.

Your ethnic background In the United States, 21% of postmenopausal women who have osteoporosis are Caucasian or Asian, 16% are Hispanic, and 10% are African American.

Black women with osteoporosis tend to be older than their white counterparts. There are several factors that may account for this difference. At skeletal maturity, and even as children, black women have more bone mass. (They also tend to have larger muscles. Muscle mass and bone mass are related; the larger the muscles, the greater the stress on the bones and the larger the bones. This might be the key.)

They also seem to lose bone at a slower rate as they get older. This is probably due to hormonal differences between races. There is evidence to suggest, for example, that blacks have higher levels of the hormone calcitonin, which helps preserve bone.

In a University of Florida survey, only 11% of women hospitalized for hip fractures were black, and they were much older than the white women who had hip fractures.

An Auburn University study showed that black women tend to lose less calcium in their urine than white women.

If you are a black woman, you can withstand more bone loss before reaching the fracture-prone state. (If your ovaries were removed at an early age, however, your risk may be nearly the same as for your white counterpart, though you have some protection because you started with more bone.)

Studies of other ethnic groups have been less extensive.

Your bone structure   If you are petite and have the same rate of bone loss as a larger woman, you will reach the fracture-prone state first, simply because you started with less bone.

How to determine the size of your bones: Extend one arm and bend the forearm upwards at a 90° angle. Keep your fingers straight and turn the inside of your wrist toward your body. Place the thumb and index finger of your other hand on the two prominent bones on either side of your elbow. Measure the space between your fingers (elbow breadth) with a ruler. (For a more accurate measurement, ask your doctor to measure your elbow breadth with calipers.)

Now find your height on the table below and read across until

HEIGHT (in 1-inch heels)	ELBOW BREADTH		
	SMALL FRAME	MEDIUM FRAME	LARGE FRAME
4'10"– 4'11"	under 2 1/4"	2 1/4"– 2 1/2"	over 2 1/2"
5'0" – 5'3"	under 2 1/4"	2 1/4"– 2 1/2"	over 2 1/2"
5'4" – 5'7"	under 2 3/8"	2 3/8"– 2 5/8"	over 2 5/8"
5'8" – 5'11"	under 2 3/8"	2 3/8"– 2 5/8"	over 2 5/8"
6'0"	under 2 1/2"	2 1/2"– 2 3/4"	over 2 3/4"

you find your elbow breadth, which will indicate whether your bone structure is small, medium, or large.

Your age at menarche   The age you start menstruating (your *menarche*) affects your bone mass at skeletal maturity. How? Bone density increases markedly during puberty, fueled by the estrogen produced by your ovaries after

Girls who start menstruating when they're older are at a higher risk for osteoporosis.

menstruation begins. So women who begin menstruating late—after the age of 16, for example—do not have the bone-building effects of estrogen for as long as those whose menarche began around age 11 or 12.

Your age at menopause   Because of the rapid bone loss that follows menopause, women who have an early menopause lose the protective effects of estrogen earlier than those whose menopause begins when they are older. For most women, the end of menstruation and reproductive capacity occurs around age 50.

LIFESTYLE

Lifestyle risk factors can contribute to loss of bone, but they are less likely, in themselves, to cause osteoporosis. It would still be wise to try to control as many as you can. This is especially important if you also have hereditary risk factors.

Poor eating habits   Normal bone development in childhood and early adulthood depends on proper nutrition. Poor eating habits can accelerate the rate of bone loss and prevent normal bone development

What you can do. Instilling good habits in your children is an important starting point. Studies have shown that adolescents who take calcium supplements significantly increase their bone

A child's poor eating habits can lead to bone loss.

mass. But, just when a teenage girl's daily calcium requirement goes up to 1,300 milligrams, her calcium intake is likely to go down. Poor dietary habits—soda pop instead of milk, potato chips instead of vegetables, for example—are a major source of the problem. Chronic dieting is another.

Other risk factors relating to eating habits include having too many of the "bone robbers": excess sodium, protein, fiber, oxalates, phytates, etc. These are described in Chapter 6.

Sedentary lifestyle Astronauts lose large amounts of calcium from their bones during only a short space flight. The reason? Restricted movement in a gravity-free environment. Similar changes occur when persons are confined to a wheelchair or bed rest for as little as several weeks.

In a study of healthy college students, it was found that it took 3 to 4 hours a day of standing or walking to counteract bone loss associated with 20 hours of bed rest.

Clearly, you either use your bones or you lose them. Some scientists believe that age-related bone loss is not inevitable, but is related to a decline in physical activity.

At the University of Pittsburgh, Jane Cauley, PhD, and her colleagues found that women who spend less than an hour a day on their feet had a substantially increased risk of hip fracture.

What you can do. Regular exercise is absolutely critical for development and maintenance of strong, healthy bones. This is true for everyone, from the developing child to the older woman. Exercise is believed to be the only non-medicinal measure that not only halts bone loss but actually stimulates the formation of new bone.

Exercise can halt bone loss and stimulate the formation of new bone.

So get up and get moving! Do something—do anything—but gradually increase your level of physical activity.

- Use the stairs instead of the elevator.
- Take a 15-minute walk during your lunch break.
- Park your car a few blocks from your destination.
- Get off the bus a few blocks before your designated stop and walk the rest of the way.

Aim for a total of 30 minutes of increased physical activity a day—for example, 15 minutes of housework in the morning and a 15-minute walk in the evening. And if you are bedridden for any length of time, take extra calcium. Dr. Robert Heaney suggests asking your doctor about increasing calcium to 2,000 mg per day for a period four times as long as you spent in bed.

Smoking Numerous studies have associated cigarette smoking with an increased risk of developing osteoporosis.

In a group of women with osteoporosis, 94% were smokers; 88% of them smoked more than a pack a day.

A Tufts University study found that postmenopausal women who smoked cigarettes had an accelerated rate of bone loss.

In a group of 72 women who had vertebral fractures from osteoporosis, 76% smoked; 68% were heavy smokers.

Menopause and its associated bone loss occurs an average of 2 years earlier in smokers than nonsmokers.

In one study, loss of bone mass was related to the number of cigarettes: nonsmokers had the most bone mass, and women who smoked half a pack daily had greater bone mass than those who smoked a whole pack.

Cigarette smoking decreases estrogen production and affects the liver's metabolism of estrogen. There's also evidence that it inhibits the growth of bone-building osteoblasts and interferes with calcium absorption.

Healing of injuries is slowed by smoking because it interrupts collagen production. Collagen is the fibrous substance the body manufactures to patch wounds and broken bones.

In a 1992 study of patients with leg bone surgery, nonsmokers regained full use of their injured legs six months earlier than smokers.

What you can do. We recommend that you make every effort

to give up this life-threatening habit. Smoking results in an increased risk of lung cancer, the leading cause of cancer death among women, and an increased risk of heart disease, the leading cause of death among women over age 40.

Plenty of help is available from community hospitals, major health organizations such as the American Cancer Society, American Heart Association and American Lung Association (look in the phone book for a local affili-

Smoking may reduce the bone mass built up earlier.

ate), and your doctor, who can help ease physical withdrawal symptoms by prescribing such products as nicotine-laced chewing gum or a nicotine skin patch. If you can't seem to quit altogether, at least cut back, and increase your intake of calcium.

Drinking Alcohol impairs calcium absorption through the intestines and it may affect the liver's ability to activate vitamin D, both of which can lead to bone loss. Severe osteoporosis has been seen in male alcoholics in their 20s. (Undoubtedly the inadequate nutrition, limited physical activity and liver damage of many alcoholics also contribute to their rapid bone loss.)

Even moderate drinking has been found to interfere with the bone remodeling cycle, reduce thickness of trabecular bone and interfere with proper bone mineralization.

Some studies have demonstrated that having as few as three drinks per day on a regular basis contributes to low bone mass.

If your bone mass is already low, there is another reason that alcohol is potentially dangerous: even a small amount can affect your balance, making you more likely to fall and sustain a fracture.

What you can do. We suggest limiting yourself to no more than one or two drinks per day. (One standard drink = 12 oz beer, 5 oz wine, or 1.5 oz of 80 proof liquor; all supply about the same amount of alcohol). Try to avoid any alcohol within an hour or two of eating calcium-rich foods or taking a calcium supplement. If you have low bone mass, try to avoid alcohol altogether.

PREGNANCY AND BREASTFEEDING

Pregnancy *For every child, a tooth.* This old saying, which can apply to bones as well as teeth, does not need to be so. It's true that a diet low in calcium during pregnancy can harm the mother's skeleton. What little calcium she takes in goes straight to the developing baby to build its bones. And if her dietary calcium is not enough to meet the needs of the fetus, the calcium reserves of her skeleton are used as well.

But pregnancy can also benefit bone mass. During pregnancy, estrogen levels are high. That stimulates the activation of vitamin D, which promotes calcium absorption and increases the production of calcitonin, which inhibits bone breakdown. Progesterone also increases dramatically during pregnancy, and this, too, has a bone-conserving effect.

> In one group of American women with osteoporosis, two-thirds had never had children.

Not enough research has been done to say whether five pregnancies, for example, are more protective than one pregnancy. All we can say conclusively is that your risk of developing osteoporosis is higher if you have had no children.

Breastfeeding Breast milk contains a lot of calcium, and the calcium has to come from somewhere. It appears that at least some of it comes from the the mother's bones. Various studies of nursing mothers have shown bone losses ranging from 6.5% to 15% over the course of several months. Not surprisingly, bone loss is more likely in women who don't get enough calcium in their diet.

What you can do. We believe that breast milk is so beneficial to babies in the first year of life that it is worth the effort to get enough calcium and vitamin D so you can breastfeed without bone loss. Most doctors advise nursing mothers to continue taking their prenatal supplements, in addition to extra calcium and vitamin D.

If you are breastfeeding and have major risk factors for osteoporosis, such as a family history, you should consider having your bone density monitored during this period. If tests reveal that you are losing bone, you may want to limit breastfeeding to the baby's first 6 months.

Case report: Lynn, age 29

Lynn had been breastfeeding her firstborn for three months when she experienced a vertebral fracture. While lifting the baby out of the crib, she fractured her 12th thoracic vertebra. Unaware that there was any relationship between breastfeeding and the fracture, she continued to nurse the baby until he was a year old.

A few years later, Lynn gave birth to her second child, whom she also breastfed. And again, as she was lifting her baby out of the crib, she fractured two more vertebrae.

This second series of fractures prompted Lynn's visit to our clinic, where she had a complete osteoporosis evaluation. We learned that Lynn's grandmother had fractured her hip, indicating a family history of osteoporosis. A physical examination revealed mild scoliosis, another risk factor.

Because Lynn had heard that calcium was important in preventing osteoporosis, she was taking calcium supplements: over 3,000 milligrams per day! She didn't know that too much calcium can actually slow down the bone remodeling cycle.

Bone density tests revealed that while Lynn's hip was normal, the density of her 4th lumbar vertebra was just 64% of peak bone mass. (It is likely that Lynn, who already had osteoporosis, lost even more bone mass while she was breastfeeding.)

To help stabilize the bone mass in her spine, we prescribed etidronate, a drug that slows bone loss. We also advised her to reduce calcium intake to 1,500 mg/day and suggested that she take low-dose oral contraceptives.

MEDICAL CONDITIONS

Several medical conditions are associated with an increased risk of osteoporosis. Most of them are chronic problems.

Diabetes   Insulin-dependent (juvenile-onset) diabetes increases your risk of developing osteoporosis, particularly if the diabetes has been poorly controlled or has been treated with large doses of insulin. Adult-onset diabetes, on the other hand, may actually be protective.

In a study from the University of California at San Diego, women with adult-onset diabetes had higher bone density of the wrist, hip and spine than those without diabetes. These women may be protected because they are generally overweight.

Arthritis   Arthritis is a degenerative disease of the joints and connective tissues characterized by inflammation, pain, and difficulty moving affected joints. There are two major types of arthritis: *osteoarthritis* and *rheumatoid arthritis*.

Some studies have suggested that women with severe rheumatoid arthritis are more likely to have osteoporosis than non-arthritic women of the same age. The reasons for this relationship are not clear. Undoubtedly, long-term treatment with corticosteroids is part of the problem, as these drugs are known to cause osteoporosis. But even those who never used corticosteroids were found to have lower bone mass than non-arthritic women.

Rheumatoid arthritis often improves with estrogen-progestogen therapy.

If there is any relationship between the two conditions, it may be related to prostaglandins, growth factors, and other substances that are formed in both conditions. Interestingly, rheumatoid arthritis often improves with postmenopausal HRT.

Many people confuse osteoporosis with arthritis. Though "osteoarthritis" sounds similar to "osteoporosis," the similarity between the two conditions ends there. In osteoarthritis, cartilage and other tissues in the joint break down, making the joints less able to move freely. *But neither bone tissue nor bone mass is affected.* Osteoarthritis is not osteoporosis.

Menstrual irregularities   Irregular menstrual cycles and cessation of menstruation *(amenorrhea)* during your reproductive years are indicators of premature bone loss. A normal menstrual cycle lasts 21 to 32 days, with an average of about 28 days. Menstrual irregularities are usually a sign of *anovulation*—a cycle in which the ovaries do not release an egg.

Stress, extreme weight changes, thyroid problems, and excessive physical exercise (training for a marathon, for example) can all cause spotting, light bleeding or missed periods. And except for pregnancy (when high estrogen levels help protect bone), anovulation is often accompanied by low estrogen and/or progesterone and accelerated bone loss similar to that of postmenopausal women.

What you can do. Any change in your cycle or menstrual blood flow can have many different underlying causes. Among them are hormone imbalances that can result in bone loss. See your doctor, who will give you a medical examination to determine the cause of the problem. If you miss a period altogether, you will be checked for pregnancy, thyroid problems or, depending on your age, your menopausal status. A pelvic exam will be done to check for ovarian cysts or other pelvic masses.

If you are found to have a low estrogen or progesterone level, you should consider having a bone density test to see if you are losing bone. If you are, you should begin treatment right away because the first years of bone loss are the most rapid.

If you have an eating disorder, you should seek professional treatment for it. Be sure to increase your calcium intake or take a calcium supplement to help ward off bone loss.

If you exercise so long and strenuously that you experience menstrual irregularities or stop menstruating, it might be a good idea to cut back on your training. You should also consider taking birth control pills, since the estrogen and progestogen in the pills help protect your bones. And you definitely should increase your calcium intake to 1,400 mg per day and take a multivitamin that contains 400 IU of vitamin D.

Some bone loss may be reversed if medical intervention begins within the first two years after exercise-induced menstrual irregularities begin. The following study suggests that some of the bone loss may be permanent.

Barbara Drinkwater, PhD, found that when amenorrheic athletes cut back on their activity level and began menstruating again, they gained 6% in spinal bone mass

over the first 15 months, the next year the increase slowed
to 3% and then stopped altogether for the next two years.

Hysterectomy   Hysterectomy—surgical removal of the
uterus—is one of the most frequently performed operations that
women have. Still, many women are confused about what it is.

Strictly speaking, hysterectomy means removal of the uterus.
A "total" or "complete" hysterectomy is removal of the uterus and
cervix. When the ovaries are also removed, the procedure is called
a *hysterectomy with oophorectomy.*

Premenopausal women who have had a hysterectomy but
retain their ovaries are not considered
to be menopausal; their ovaries still produce hormones. Even so, many of them
have significantly lower bone density of
the hip and spine than menstruating women of the same age.

Sometimes the ovaries stop producing hormones after a hysterectomy.

Some researchers have reported that in about one-
third of the women who have had a hysterectomy, the
ovaries cease to function within one to two years after
surgery. These women may actually experience a surgically
induced, gradual menopause.

Hysterectomy with oophorectomy. Some physicians routinely recommend hysterectomy with oophorectomy, particularly for
women who are near menopause age. They reason that since the
patient can no longer have children and the ovaries will lose their
function at menopause anyway, the surgery will prevent the possibility of ovarian cancer developing at a later date. Ovarian cancer
is not common, but when it does occur, it is often fatal.

If you had both ovaries removed before your natural menopause ("surgical menopause") you are no longer getting estrogen
from the ovaries. The younger you were when you had surgery,
the more years you have not had estrogen to protect your bones.
Surgical menopause increases your risk of osteoporosis by 50%.

What you can do. Most hysterectomies are "elective," which
means they are performed to treat conditions for which there are
other treatment alternatives. If you do not have a life-threatening

condition (such as cancer), you should discuss all of your options with your doctor before consenting to the surgery.

While the logic of removing the ovaries at the time of hysterectomy may at first appear sound, it must be placed in perspective. The chances of developing ovarian cancer range from 1 in 1,000 to 14 in 1,000, depending on which study you look at. By comparison, breast cancer affects 1 in 9 women and colon cancer affects 1 in 22. (How many physicians recommend removal of these organs as a means of preventing future cancer?)

Moreover, earlier diagnosis of ovarian cancer is becoming more feasible thanks to ultrasound, which has become an important diagnostic tool for women with a suspicious pelvic mass. A blood test that detects levels of CA-125, a substance produced by ovarian tumors, used with ultrasound to determine the nature of the pelvic mass, can help determine whether or not an ovarian mass is cancerous.

Osteoporosis, on the other hand, is known to occur at a relatively early age in one-fourth to one-half of women who have had both ovaries removed prior to a natural menopause, if they do not receive postmenopausal hormones. You will have to decide if preventing unlikely ovarian cancer outweighs the very real risk of osteoporosis.

Discuss the pros and cons of leaving your ovaries alone if they are healthy and if you have no family history of ovarian cancer. If they must be removed, discuss how you will go about preventing the rapid bone loss that follows a surgical menopause.

Scoliosis   Research has suggested that the S-shaped curvature of the spine known as scoliosis—or the risk factors associated with scoliosis—may place women at a greater risk of developing osteoporosis.

In 50 women with osteoporosis, half of them had a 10° or higher curvature of the spine. (Spinal fractures did not cause the curvature.) The researchers noted that when such women are treated by surgical fusion of the spine, weak, osteoporotic bone is usually found.

Researchers who studied 75 ballet dancers found a possible association between scoliosis and increased risk of fractures. But those with scoliosis often had other risk factors, such as late menarche (after age 14) and irregular menstrual cycles: the dancers with the most fractures (usually stress fractures in the toes) were twice as likely to have had temporary amenorrhea (cessation of menstruation) than dancers who suffered few or no fractures.

The presence of scoliosis on physical examination is an important sign of latent or potential osteoporosis. Most public schools now offer routine screening for scoliosis. If you have never had your back examined for evidence of scoliosis, this may be a good time.

Gastric surgery   Women who have had part of their stomach removed because of cancer or severe ulcers are at greater risk because they are less able to absorb calcium from their food. The same is true of women who have had gastric bypass surgery for the treatment of obesity.

Endocrine disorders   Certain endocrine (hormonal) disorders have been associated with a high risk of osteoporosis:

Hyperparathyroidism. Parathyroid hormone helps regulate blood calcium levels, in part by releasing calcium from the bones. When excessive amounts of this hormone are excreted from the parathyroid glands, higher-than-normal blood calcium levels result. One of the consequences of this disease, if left untreated, is rapid bone loss.

Hyperthyroidism. Overactivity of the thyroid gland can lead to an accelerated rate of bone breakdown and loss of bone mass. Likewise, women who take excessive amounts of thyroid medication for treatment of an *underactive* thyroid (hypothyroidism) are also at greater risk of bone loss.

Hyperprolactinemia is characterized by an increased blood level of *prolactin* (hormone involved in breast milk production, secreted by the pituitary gland). Women with the condition often stop menstruating and have estrogen levels as low as those of post-menopausal women. It is accompanied by rapid bone loss.

Cushing's syndrome occurs when the adrenal glands produce too much cortisol. Adrenal hormones inhibit osteoblasts and make the bones more susceptible to the bone-dissolving effects of para-thyroid hormone, leading to excessive bone loss.

Lactose intolerance If you cannot drink milk or even have an ice cream cone without suffering from gas, stomach cramps or diarrhea, you may have *lactose intolerance*, a lack of the intestinal enzyme *lactase*. Lactose is a sugar found in milk and other dairy products; lactase metabolizes lactose into easily digested fractions.

This common problem affects 21% of whites, 51% of hispanics and 80% of African-Americans in the U.S. It also affects a high proportion of Asians, Eskimos, Native Americans and South Americans. It is more prevalent in the elderly.

Among white women, lactose intolerance is nine times more prevalent in those who have osteoporosis. The likely cause is that women who stop eating dairy products generally do not replace them with other calcium sources. So **Lactose insufficiency is nine times more prevalent in white women with osteoporosis.** what begins as a lactase deficiency develops into a calcium deficiency.

In black women, the high incidence of lactose intolerance coupled with their low incidence of osteoporosis suggests that ethnic protection overrides the risk associated with the lactase—and calcium—deficiency.

What you can do. You may be able to tolerate small to moderate amounts of dairy products, particularly if they are part of a meal. Yogurt is better tolerated than milk, especially yogurt with active cultures, and yogurt cheese is even better because it has about half the lactose of yogurt. Whole milk causes fewer problems than skim because fat slows the rate of stomach emptying. Hard cheese has most of the lactose removed when it is made.

You can add lactase drops to milk. You may want to try lactose-reduced milk (Lactaid, Dairy Ease). Adding the drops to lactose-reduced milk will remove nearly all the lactose.

Eating disorders   Women with the eating disorders *bulimia* and *anorexia* see themselves as "too fat," even though they are typically of normal weight or even underweight. Bulimic women go on uncontrollable eating binges, followed by self-induced vomiting or the use of laxatives or diuretics. Anorexic women eat so little that they literally starve themselves.

Either one of these eating disorders can permanently retard bone metabolism. There are multiple reasons that such women have lower bone mass than other women of the same age. One is inadequate calcium. Anorexic women eat so little that profound nutritional deficiencies occur; in bulimic women, laxatives and diuretics may interfere with calcium absorption. Both groups have menstrual irregularities. Anorexic women usually stop menstruating for months or even years. More than 40% of bulimic women stop menstruating or have irregular menstrual cycles. Menopause may occur prematurely. In some, bone loss is so severe that fractures occur long before the menopausal years.

What you can do. Admitting that you have a problem may be the hardest step you take toward recovery. Treatment generally lasts one to two years and requires a team approach by trained professionals, including a physician, nutrition counselor and psychologist or psychiatrist. The earlier that treatment is begun, the more successful it is likely to be and the sooner associated bone loss can be stopped.

Broken bones   As noted in Chapter 1, if you've had even one fracture, it's a sign of a weakened skeleton, and your risk of another fracture is greatly increased.

DRUGS

A number of medications are associated with bone loss. Some may interfere with bone remodeling or calcium absorption. Others merely aggravate an existing tendency to bone loss. Together with your physician, you may be able to reassess your need for certain medications, perhaps changing to a lower dose or to an alternative. If neither of these is possible, you will need to be especially attentive to protecting your bones with diet and exercise and, where relevant,

take antiresorptive therapy (such as HRT, one of the bisphosphonates, or the recently approved SERM drugs).

Heparin   If you need to be on prolonged anticoagulant therapy, you may be able to switch to a coumadin-type alternative.

Corticosteroids   These drugs are often used to ameliorate
symptoms of osteo- and rheumatoid arthri-
tis, asthma, lupus and glaucoma. The most   **Osteoporosis from steroids is**
common corticosteroids are *cortisone,*   **more severe than post-**
hydrocortisone, prednisone and *dexam-*   **menopausal osteoporosis.**
ethasone. They appear to induce bone loss
by decreasing calcium absorption, increasing calcium excretion, and
suppressing formation of new bone. Steroid-induced osteoporosis
is characterized by loss of bone from the ribs and subsequent rib fractures. It is much more severe than postmenopausal osteoporosis.

If you have arthritis, you may be able to achieve similar relief
with one of the nonsteroidal anti-inflammatory drugs, such as Advil,
Naprosyn or Relafen.

Insulin   If you need insulin for diabetes, there may be ways
to reduce the amount. Losing weight is one possibility. Another
is exercise.

There is also a new class of oral drugs that enhances the tissue metabolism of insulin, thus permitting lower doses of injected
insulin to achieve and maintain good blood-glucose control. Drug cat-
egories include metformin (Glucophage) and troglitazide (Precose).

Thyroid medication   High doses of thyroid supplements are
believed to produce a physiological state
similar to that of thyroid gland overactivity   **An overactive thyroid is a**
(hyperthyroidism), which is known to in-   **risk factor. So is medication**
crease the risk of osteoporosis.   **for an underactive thyroid.**

Studies have found that women taking supplements
equivalent to or greater than 3 grains of dessicated thyroid (or 300 micrograms of lethothyroxine) had significantly lower bone mass than other women.

Premenopausal women who had taken thyroid supplements for more than five years had a 10% lower bone density of the hip than women of the same age who had never taken them.

You can take a blood test to determine your level of thyroid-stimulating hormone (TSH), a pituitary hormone that stimulates the thyroid gland when thyroid hormones fall below normal levels. If TSH is low, you may be taking more thyroid than you need, and your doctor can adjust the dosage.

Anticonvulsants   Anticonvulsant drugs such as *phenytoin, phenobarbital, primidone* and *phensuximide* are metabolized in the liver. There, they stimulate production of enzymes that break down vitamin D, leading to a vitamin D deficiency and, indirectly, to a calcium deficiency (since vitamin D is needed for calcium absorption). The result is bone loss due to both osteomalacia (from the vitamin D deficiency) and osteoporosis (from the calcium deficiency).

Antacids   Women constitute an increasing number of the estimated 2.5 million Americans with newly diagnosed ulcers. They, along with many others who do not have ulcer problems, are daily users of antacids, over-the-counter products that seem harmless.

But many antacids contain aluminum, which can increase calcium excretion. This calcium comes from the bones. Sometimes one risk factor is related to another, as when people on corticosteroids have gastrointestinal symptoms and take antacids to alleviate them.

If you are taking an antacid that contains aluminum, you may be able to cut back on its use and deal with your gastrointestinal problems through dietary and behavior modification. If not, switch to one that does not contain aluminum.

Aluminum-containing antacids can lead to bone loss.

Antacids containing aluminum: Amphojel, Delcid, Di-Gel, Gaviscon, Gelusil, Maalox, Mylanta, Riopan.

Antacids without aluminum: Alka-Selzer, Alka-2, Bisodol, Citrocarbonate, Eno, Marblen, Percy Medicine, Rolaids, Titralac, Tums.

Some antacids, such as Tums and Rolaids, contain calcium and can actually double as calcium supplements. If you are not sure about your antacid, look on the label or ask your pharmacist.

Diuretics Diuretics promote the production of urine and are often prescribed for people with high blood pressure. In terms of their effects on calcium balance and bone mass, some diuretics are good and some are bad.

- *Furosemide* (e.g., Lasix) increases urinary calcium excretion.

- *Thiazide* (e.g., HCTZ) reduces the amount of calcium lost in urine and has been shown to *increase* bone mass.

If you are taking a furosemide-type diuretic, it may be a good idea to change to a thiazide type.

Gonatropin releasing hormone agonists These drugs (Lupron, Synarel)—used to treat gynecological problems such as endometriosis, fibroid tumors of the uterus and severe premenstrual syndrome (PMS)—reduce estrogen and progesterone levels in the body. The result is a rapid loss of bone mass similar to that of postmenopausal women. Hormone levels return to normal when the drug is stopped.

If you need these drugs for more than six months, your doctor will likely prescribe estrogen/progestogen add-back therapy to protect your bones.

PROTECTIVE FACTORS

Contraception Birth control pills, in addition to being one of the most effective forms of reversible contraception available, can protect your bones because they contain estrogen and progestogen, hormones that inhibits bone breakdown.

Robert Lindsay, MD, PhD, and his colleagues at Columbia University found that long-time users of oral contraceptives had stronger bones than those who had never taken them. At least two other major studies have confirmed these findings.

Women on oral contraceptives for at least eight years had bone mass that was 12% higher; each year, density of the spine increased by about 1%. Overall, 82% had higher-than-average bone density for their age.

Oral contraceptives also offer other health benefits, including protection against ovarian cysts, ovarian cancer, endometrial cancer, benign cysts of the breast, iron-deficiency anemia and pelvic inflammatory disease (bacterial infection of the reproductive tract).

What are the risks? Because today's oral contraceptives contain much less estrogen and progestogen than those prescribed in the 1960s and 1970s, they are safer. Most of the research conducted to date has found no increased risk of breast cancer associated with their use. There is no increase in heart attacks.

Blood clots (the kind that can precipitate a stroke) occasionally develop. We suspect that platelets (blood cells that help form a clot) may somehow be affected by estrogen. Women over age 35 can counteract this effect by taking one junior aspirin (81 mg) every 3 days. Aspirin decreases the stickiness of platelets and protects against spasm of the coronary arteries, which could trigger a heart attack. *Check with your doctor before taking aspirin regularly. Even though it's sold over-the-counter, some people should not take aspirin.*

Why not use postmenopausal estrogens, which contain one-sixth the estrogen of oral contaceptives and are known to protect bone? There are several reasons: they do not contain enough estrogen to protect against unwanted pregnancy; you may require more estrogen to protect your bones than postmenopausal women; and the progestogen in oral contraceptives offers added protection against bone loss.

Your weight   If you are more than 30% over your ideal body weight, you are less likely to develop osteoporosis. Before menopause, the ovaries produce large amounts of estrogen and progesterone, and smaller amounts of **Body fat reduces your risk of osteoporosis.** androgens, the male sex hormones. The adrenal glands also produce androgens. After menopause, production of estrogen and progesterone drops drastically, but the amount of androgens stays about the same.

These androgens are chemically converted to estrogen in fat tissue. The more fat you have, the more estrogen you can produce. Fat, therefore, substantially reduces your risk of osteoporosis. But for the same reason, you have an increased risk of breast cancer and a three- to ninefold increased risk of uterine cancer. The risk of developing cancer of the uterine lining (an estrogen-dependent cancer) exists because the ovaries are no longer producing progesterone, which normally protects the uterus from estrogen over-stimulation.

What you can do. First, consider having a bone density test, to find out if you are losing bone. Talk to your doctor about having a "progesterone challenge test," which will determine if you are producing an excessive amount of estrogen. If you are, you may need to be taking a progestogen to protect your uterus.

Case report: Jean, age 32

Many women with major risk factors never develop osteoporosis, while others with no risk factors, do. Jean is a perfect example of a woman who appears to be at little or no risk.

Jean came to our clinic to participate in a weight loss program. At 5'6" and 226 pounds, she had a serious weight problem, but was otherwise healthy.

A total body scan using dual-energy x-ray absorptiometry (DEXA) was done to determine Jean's percentage of body fat. The test also uncovered that her bone density was 15% below that of the average woman at skeletal maturity. This was not expected because she had none of the risk factors for osteoporosis, and in addition her weight should have protected her.

Fortunately, the problem was caught in plenty of time to help prevent serious bone loss. We recommended that Jean increase her calcium intake through food and supplements and also exercise regularly, both to lose weight and build bone.

Fluoride   People who drink fluoridated water have stronger bones than those who don't. But what if your water isn't fluoridated? Should you be taking fluoride supplements? The answer is no,

RISK FACTOR ASSESSMENT I

Each "yes" answer ***increases*** your risk of osteoporosis

REPRODUCTIVE STATUS

First period at age 16 or older	☐ Yes	☐ No
Irregular periods prior to menopause	☐ Yes	☐ No
Never been pregnant	☐ Yes	☐ No
Natural menopause before age 40	☐ Yes	☐ No
Ovaries removed before age 40	☐ Yes	☐ No
Five or more years since menopause	☐ Yes	☐ No

FRACTURE HISTORY

Family history of osteoporosis	☐ Yes	☐ No
Loss of height *(more than 1")*	☐ Yes	☐ No
Spontaneous fractures *(no trauma)*	☐ Yes	☐ No

MEDICAL HISTORY

Rheumatoid arthritis	☐ Yes	☐ No
Overactive thyroid	☐ Yes	☐ No
Parathyroid disease	☐ Yes	☐ No
Gastrectomy *(removal of stomach)*	☐ Yes	☐ No
Chronic kidney disease	☐ Yes	☐ No
Periodontal gum disease	☐ Yes	☐ No
Chronic diarrhea	☐ Yes	☐ No
Lactose intolerance	☐ Yes	☐ No
Eating disorder (anorexia nervosa or bulimia)	☐ Yes	☐ No

MEDICATIONS TAKEN FOR ONE YEAR OR MORE

Diuretics *(furosemides)*	☐ Yes	☐ No
Anticonvulsants	☐ Yes	☐ No
Cortisone	☐ Yes	☐ No
Antacids that contain aluminum	☐ Yes	☐ No
Thyroid medication	☐ Yes	☐ No

DAILY LIFESTYLE

Don't exercise	☐ Yes	☐ No
Cigarettes: more than 1 pack	☐ Yes	☐ No
Caffeine: more than 5 cups coffee, tea, cola	☐ Yes	☐ No
Alcohol: more than 2 drinks	☐ Yes	☐ No
Low calcium diet	☐ Yes	☐ No

RISK FACTOR ASSESSMENT II

Each "yes" answer **decreases** your risk of osteoporosis

REPRODUCTIVE STATUS

First period at age 11–12	☐ Yes	☐ No
Regular periods prior to menopause	☐ Yes	☐ No
One or more pregnancies	☐ Yes	☐ No
Natural menopause at age 50 or older	☐ Yes	☐ No

FRACTURE HISTORY

No family history of osteoporosis	☐ Yes	☐ No
Same height	☐ Yes	☐ No
Have never had spontaneous fractures	☐ Yes	☐ No

MEDICATIONS TAKEN FOR ONE YEAR OR MORE

Birth control pills	☐ Yes	☐ No
Hormone therapy	☐ Yes	☐ No

DAILY LIFESTYLE

Exercise	☐ Yes	☐ No
Dairy products	☐ Yes	☐ No
Calcium supplements	☐ Yes	☐ No

---

although fluoride is being investigated as a bone-building treatment for women with low bone mass or established osteoporosis.

SIGNS OF BONE LOSS

There are some tell-tale signs of bone loss you should be aware of. By the time one of these is identified, it is very likely that your bones have already become seriously weakened or damaged. Your best protection is to have a bone density test right away (*see Chapter 5*) and if you appear to be losing bone mass, discuss ways of stopping bone loss and increasing bone mass with your doctor.

Loss of height The most obvious sign of osteoporosis is loss of height. Since the bones of your legs do not become shorter, all the height is lost between your hips and neck.

The simplest way to determine whether you have lost height is to compare your present height with your height at age 20. If you do not know exactly how tall you were then, you can make an estimate by measuring your arm span, since during that period arm span and height are nearly equal.

Hold your arms straight out to the sides and have someone measure from fingertips to fingertips. Now subtract your head-to-heel height from your arm span. This will give you a rough indication of height loss.

A good way to monitor your height in the years ahead is to measure your crown-to-rump height. Sit on a chair and have someone measure the distance from the top of your head to the bottom of your spine. This can be done by your physician at your annual physical examination or at home by a family member.

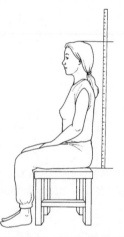

CROWN-TO-RUMP HEIGHT

Transparent skin   Look at the back of your hand. Is the skin loose and lacking in pigmentation? Can you see the edges of both the large and small veins? If the answer is yes, you are also probably over the age of 60, since younger women seldom have transparent skin.

In 1941 Fuller Albright, MD, the physician credited with first linking osteoporosis and menopause, noted that many of his osteoporotic patients had transparent skin.

One formal study of older women with osteoporosis showed that 83% had transparent skin on the backs of their hands.

Your doctor can measure your skin thickness with calipers that pinch the skin on the back of the hand and pull it away from the underlying tissues. There is very little fat in this area, so the findings will be the same whether you are fat or thin.

Using this technique, scientists have found that opaque skin is 35% thicker than transparent skin. Most noticeable on the back of the hand, the transparency is due to a lack of collagen in the skin's outer layers. Since collagen is also a major component of bone, it is reasonable to conclude that "thin skin" is associated with "thin bones."

So far, the technique has not been proven reliable enough for use as a predictor of osteoporosis. This may soon change. Researchers in the United Kingdom, using x-ray techniques, have found a correlation between skin collagen in the hand and bone density. More objective tests of skin thickness based on this technology are now in the works.

Periodontal disease   Periodontal disease (perio = around, dontal = teeth), sometimes called pyorrhea, is a condition involving the supporting tissues of the teeth: the gums, the ligaments attaching teeth to the jawbone, and sometimes the jawbone itself. It is a major cause of tooth loss in adults, appears most often in the middle years, and is more common in women than men.

Dentists have known for years that loss of bone in the jaw often accompanies periodontal disease. But like the chicken-and-egg puzzler, it's still not clear whether periodontal disease causes bone loss or vice versa. Some studies have found a correlation between tooth loss and bone loss elsewhere in the body, suggesting that periodontal disease may signal impending osteoporosis. But other studies, including our own, have found no increased risk. Nevertheless, bone loss in the jaw may precede and therefore warn of bone loss elsewhere in the body. And conversely, taking estrogen may help protect bone in the jaw and elsewhere.

A study of 300 women between the ages of 50 and 74 found that those taking estrogen had less bone loss around the teeth and more of their own teeth than the women not on estrogen.

Weak muscles There have been some striking correlations between muscle strength and bone mass.

In a study by Wendy C. Bevier and colleagues, grip strength was seen as a good indicator of bone density in elderly women.

Australian researcher, Nicolas Pocock, found that muscle strength in both the arms (biceps) and legs (quadriceps) could predict bone mass in the hip, spine and forearm.

This is not so surprising, since the larger the muscles, the greater the stress on the bones and the larger the bones.

Although other scientists have demonstrated that muscle strength could predict bone density in young women, it may be a while before simple tests are devised that can reliably predict bone density. But if you are concerned, your doctor or physical therapist may be able to give you a rough idea of your muscle strength.

5 How To *Know* if You Are Losing Bone

In the past, by the time bone loss was apparent to a woman or her physician, extensive and irreversible damage had already taken place. Information from the medical and family history, lifestyle and other risk factors identified only about one-third of those who had osteopenia.

Now you can actually *know* if you have osteoporosis or are at risk for it. You can take a simple bone density test that identifies small changes in bone mass long before a fracture occurs. Densitometry, as it's called, is painless, quick, easy and safe; it requires no special preparation, medication or injection; and the exposure to radiation is very low (less than a dental x-ray).

If more information is needed, special urine and blood tests can assess the rate of bone loss or bone formation. These tests, together with bone density tests, have become indispensable tools in the detection of osteopenia and in the treatment of osteoporosis.

DENSITOMETRY

Of all the tests, densitometry is the most accurate way to tell how much bone you have and whether or not you are losing bone. An

Densitometry is the most accurate measure of bone mass.

instrument called a *densitometer* measures *bone density*, the amount of bone mineral (mostly calcium) in relation to the width of the bone. It does this by calculating how many rays of a radioactive material (or x-rays) are absorbed by the bone; greater absorption = greater bone mineral content and greater bone mineral density (BMD).

To predict your fracture risk, your test results are compared with the average bone density in a large population of "young normal" women at 35, the age when women reach skeletal maturity. This is often referred to as *peak bone mass.*

Spine and hip measurements are better predictors of fracture risk than the wrist or heel. In the spine or hip, every 10% decrease

Every 10% decrease in bone density below peak bone mass doubles fracture risk.

in bone density below peak bone mass doubles a woman's risk of fracture.

Two types of densitometry are in use today: single x-ray absorptiometry (SXA) and dual-energy x-ray absorptiometry (DEXA). Their differences are in the equipment, source of radiation, and which bones are measured. Most densitometers can accurately detect a 1–2% change in bone density.

BONE MINERAL, BONE DENSITY, AND BONE MASS: WHAT'S THE DIFFERENCE?

Several terms are used to describe how much bone you have. The differences between them are subtle.

Bone mineral content —the total amount of calcium in your bones.

Bone mass—the total amount of calcium plus all the other minerals in your bones.

Bone density—the bone mineral content in relation to the width of your bones. Same as bone mineral density (BMD).

Radiation exposure: Densitometry tests have only a very small exposure, which is measured in mrems (for millirems and pronounced emrems). The DEXA test, for example, uses only 1 to 3 mrems of radiation. For comparison, a full dental x-ray is 300 mrems.

Single x-ray absorptiometry (SXA) A single beam of gamma rays is used to measure bone density of the forearm (usually the wrist) or the heel. This technique is often referred to as "peripheral densitometry" because it can only test bone density in the lower portion of the arm or leg.

A number of instruments are now available for this test; these include PIXI (Lunar Corp.), P-DEXA (Norland) and accuDEXA (Schick Technologies). All operate on the same principle. The part being measured is placed between the source of radiation and a detector. A scanner passes over the bone several times as it measures the amount of gamma rays that passes through the bone and soft tissue. The test is painless.

SXA replaces an earlier test called single photon absorptiometry (SPA). SPA utilized a radioactive isotope as the source of the gamma radiation, and the heel or forearm was placed in a water bath to keep the rays from scattering.

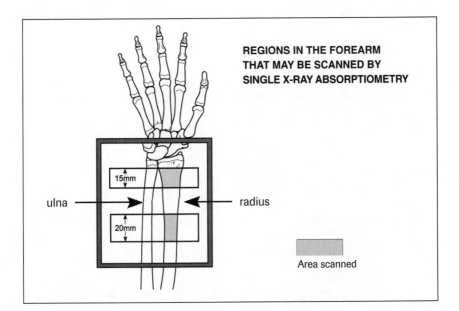

REGIONS IN THE FOREARM
THAT MAY BE SCANNED BY
SINGLE X-RAY ABSORPTIOMETRY

ulna — radius

15mm

20mm

Area scanned

How long does it take? 5 seconds for a wrist or heel scan with one of the newer machines.

Radiation exposure: 20 mrems.

Benefits: Inexpensive; good accuracy and precision; values correlate well with the bone density of the spine and hip.

Drawbacks: Cannot reliably measure the density of bones located deeper in the body, such as the hip or spinal vertebrae. Cannot determine maximal bone loss and where it is mostly found. Not suited for monitoring a bone density in response to treatment.

Best use: As a baseline test to identify women at risk for osteopenia. Those showing high bone density will be reassured; those with low or borderline values should have a DEXA test.

Dual-energy x-ray absorptiometry (DEXA, DXA)   This is considered the best and most accurate method for measuring bone density. You lie on a padded platform while a wand-like device passes over your body, measuring the density of the spine or hip.

DEXA is the most accurate test of bone density.

Spine. Although most spinal fractures occur in the thoracic vertebrae (the middle part of the spine), it is impossible to measure

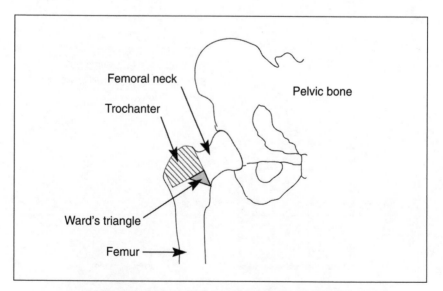

SITES FOR MEASURING BONE DENSITY OF THE HIP

bone density there because the rib cage and sternum (breastbone) get in the way. Instead, DEXA determines the density of four lumbar (lower back) vertebrae: L1, L2, L3 and L4.

Hip. Bone density of the hip is measured in three places:

(1) the *femoral neck,* actually the upper part of the thighbone;

(2) the *trochanter,* the outer part of the upper thighbone; and

(3) *Ward's triangle*, an area on the upper part of the thighbone where the femoral neck is connected to the main shaft of the bone.

DEXA replaces dual photon absorptiometry (DPA), which used two beams of gamma rays to measure the density of the hip and

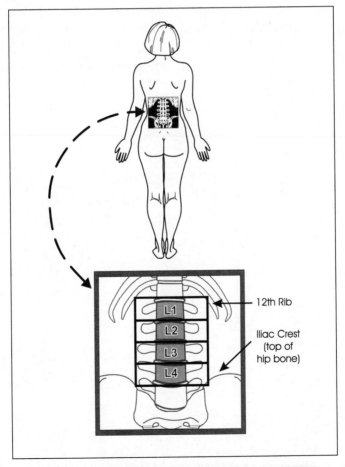

SITES FOR MEASURING BONE DENSITY OF THE SPINE

certain vertebrae. It was not ideal because the amount of radiation delivered by the radioactive isotope (gadolinium) changed as the isotope decayed, affecting the test results.

How long does it take? 3 to 7 minutes.

Radiation exposure: Almost none: only 1 to 3 mrems.

Benefits: Good accuracy and precision. A DEXA scan of the lumbar vertebrae or hip can detect even a 1% bone loss and is an excellent barometer of fracture risk.

Drawbacks: Relatively high cost, though it is approved by Medicare and covered by many insurance policies.

A potential problem is that if calcium deposits form in the body, they are included in the measurement (around an arthritic joint, for example), and could lead to an overestimation of bone mass. (Newer models of DEXA may help resolve this problem with so-called lateral testing, which assesses only the trabecular portion of the vertebrae.)

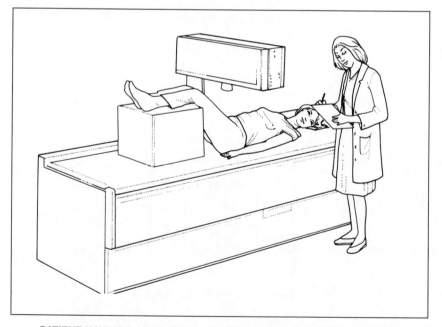

PATIENT HAVING A DEXA BONE DENSITY TEST OF THE LUMBAR SPINE

X-RAYS

For detecting early bone loss, standard x-rays are not sensitive enough to be of much practical value; even the most experienced radiologist cannot detect a problem until more than 30% of bone mass has been lost. Combined with densitometry, however, x-rays can sometimes be used for assessing the clinical impact of a low bone density test.

X-rays do not detect a problem until over 30% of bone mass has been lost.

Spinal and hip x-rays   Because x-rays of the spine or hip can detect fractures, they can help in determining how much damage has occurred. Women with low bone density and whose x-rays show a vertebral deformity are at greater risk of future fracture than women with same same amount of bone loss but normal vertebrae on x-ray. Standard x-rays can also help differentiate between osteoporosis and other causes of spinal deformities.

X-rays of the jaw   Bone loss in the jaw may precede and therefore warn of bone loss elsewhere in the body, so dentists are in a unique position to identify women at risk of osteoporosis. If x-rays of your jaw show reduced bone density, you should report this finding to your physician, who can arrange for more conclusive bone density tests.

Radiographic absorptiometry   In this test, also called *radiographic photodensitometry*, a computer scanner determines bone density from an x-ray of the hand.

A small piece of aluminum alloy, which has a known density, is placed next to the hand as the x-ray is taken. Then a computer scans the x-ray and compares the density of the bone to the density of the aluminum alloy.

Radiographic absorptiometry predicts spinal density with 90% accuracy.

How long does it take? 3 to 5 minutes.

Radiation exposure: 100 mrems.

Benefits: Needs no special equipment. Ten times more accurate than ordinary x-rays, which must be inspected visually.

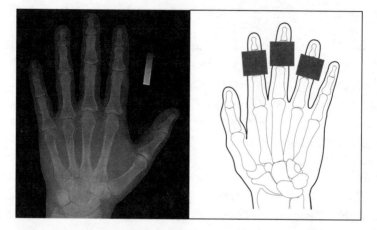

RADIOGRAPHIC ABSORPTIOMETRY. *Left:* X-ray of the hand taken with an aluminum alloy reference wedge placed next to the fingers. *Right:* Indicates the three sites bone density is measured.

Radiographic absorptiometry of the hand has been found be a good reflection of bone mass elsewhere in the body: it is 90% correct in predicting density of the lumbar spine and 82% correct in predicting density of the hip, making it a useful screening test for low bone mass in the hip and spine.

Drawbacks: As with SXA, this method cannot determine or quantify the maximum region of bone loss in the spine and hip.

CT scan   A CT (or CAT) scan is a three-dimensional view of the body created by x-rays and a computer. It can measure the exact amount of trabecular bone within an individual vertebra.

For the test, you lie on a moveable examining table inside a long hollow cylinder containing an x-ray scanner.

How long does it take? 10 to 15 minutes.

Drawbacks: Exposes your internal organs to relatively high amounts of radiation. It is expensive; it tends to overestimate the amount of bone being lost. Probably will not be used routinely for bone density scanning.

TEST	SITE	PRECISION[1]	ACCURACY[2]	EXAM TIME	RADIATION[3]	COST[4]
SXA (single x-ray absorptiometry	Wrist	1-3%	1-5%	5 sec.	20 mrems	$75
Radiographic absorptiometry	Hand	1-2%	4%	3-5 min.	100 mrems	$75-150
DEXA (dual-energy x-ray absorptiometry)	Spine, hip total body	0.5-2%	3-5%	3-7 min.	1-3 mrems	$125-200
CT scan	Spine	2-5%	5-20%	10-15 min.	100-1,000 mrems	$150-250

COMPARING THE TESTS THAT MEASURE BONE DENSITY

[1] Precision: difference between 2 tests done within 1/2 hour of each other.
[2] Accuracy: amount of bone mineral actually present in the site tested.
[3] For comparison, a chest x-ray gives 20 to 50 mrems of radiation, a full dental x-ray, 300 mrems.
[4] Approximate.

ULTRASOUND

Ultrasound involves high-frequency sound waves sent through the body's tissues. It does not use radiation. The sound waves probably measure the amount of collagen in bone, which may indirectly tell us something about the bone's elasticity, or shock-absorbability and bone strength. A decrease in elasticity has been associated with a 30 to 35% increase in the risk of osteoporosis.

Ultrasound can assess new bone formation.

Ultrasound can monitor bone collagen—and thus, new bone formation—during treatment for osteopenia or osteoporosis. (Ultrasound tests have been found to correlate with the microscopic anatomy of trabecular bone.) As a diagnostic tool, however, the technology is still being evaluated in clinical practice and although recently FDA-approved, should *not* be used as a substitute for DEXA testing. It will probably be best used in conjunction with other bone density tests.

SHOULD YOU HAVE A BONE DENSITY TEST?

Densitometry can detect osteoporosis before a break occurs, determine the rate of bone loss, and track the efficacy of any treatment you are having. If you are postmenopausal and not sure whether to begin bone conserving therapy (e.g., estrogen, Fosamax), these specialized x-rays can help you make a decision.

We recommend having your bone density tested if you have or have had any of the following:

- Early menopause (before age 40)

- Late menarche

- Surgical removal of ovaries

- Prolonged amenorrhea (cessation of menstruation)

- Family history of osteoporosis

- Small stature and slender build

- History or x-ray evidence of fractures

- Rheumatoid arthritis, hyperthyroidism, hyperparathyroidism, type I diabetes, chronic liver or kidney disease

- Regular and/or prolonged use of steroids, thyroid hormones, anticonvulsants, heparin, or chemotherapy

- An eating disorder (anorexia nervosa or bulimia)

- Diet low in calcium

- Sedentary lifestyle

- Gastric surgery

- Heavy use of alcohol or cigarettes

If you are already being treated for osteopenia or osteoporosis, a bone density test can help determine the appropriate dosage of medication and whether or not the treatment regimen is working

Another reason to be tested is to know how much your efforts are accomplishing or whether you are losing bone mass despite an appropriate exercise and lifestyle program. It serves as a kind of progress report to keep motivation high. We found, in our clinic, that women who had had a bone density test were much more likely to continue eating right and exercising regularly than those who had not had a test.

We gave 771 women over age 30 a pamphlet describing osteoporosis and its prevention. Over half of them (418) also had a bone density test. A year later, three-fourths of those who had the test had made lifestyle changes, such as increasing calcium or exercising regularly, compared to only about half of those who did not have the test.

WHEN SHOULD YOU BE TESTED?

Ideally, you would have your first assessment during your 30s or 40s, to determine how much bone you have at skeletal maturity. If your bone mass is normal, you are off to a good start. But if you find you are entering the bone-losing years with an already low bone mass, you should be particularly attentive to your diet and exercise habits and begin controlling as many risk factors *(see chapter 4)* as you can.

Your next assessment should be made soon after menopause, when the most rapid bone loss begins due to a decline in estrogen production.

- *If the test shows normal bone density:* You should consider a density test every 3–5 years, so long as you have annual urine collagen-excretion tests *(described in next section)* and they are normal. After menopause, regular assessments should continue at least until you are 75 and maybe beyond.

- *If the test shows low to low-normal density:* You should have at least two or three annual tests to determine how fast you are losing bone. If you find you are losing more than 1% of bone mass per year, try to step up preventive measures.

How often you need to be tested will be determined by how rapidly you are losing bone, how sensitive the technique is, and what prevention strategies you are using.

How available are bone density tests? To find out what is available in your community, ask your doctor or your County

HOW THE DOCTOR INTERPRETS THE RESULTS OF

Although the format of the test results may vary with the equipment used, the principle of interpreting them is the same.

The *numbers listed at the left* represent bone mineral density (BMD)—the density of mineral (calcium, phosphorus, etc.) in the specific bone tissue measured.

The white line indicates *peak bone mass* and how it changes with age (maximum is 1.20). The *range of age-matched values* (shaded area) indicates the normal range of BMD for each age. The *black dot* represents your bone density reading.

Your bone density is compared to the average bone density in a large population of "young normal" women at 35, the age at which women reach skeletal maturity ("peak bone mass"). Your bone density is given as a percentage of this group.

In the test result below, a 62-year-old woman has a bone density reading of .96, which is 80% of peak bone mass. By falling into the shaded area, her BMD is in the average range for her age, though it still indicates a moderate degree of osteopenia.

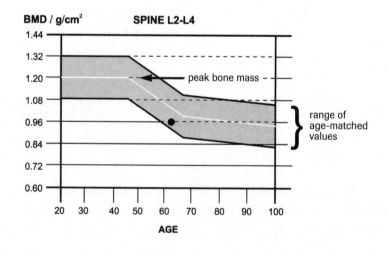

YOUR BONE DENSITY TEST

Now look at this test result, which appears to be identical to the other one. The difference is that this woman is 45 years old, which gives her an extra 20 years' exposure to further bone loss. For her, a bone density of 80% indicates a serious potential for fractures.

There is no exact dividing line between osteopenia and osteoporosis. Generally, values in the 75% to 90% range of peak bone mass are considered to be osteopenia, and values at or below 75% indicate osteoporosis. But some researchers identify osteoporosis by a fracture.

PERCENTAGE OF PEAK BONE MASS	INTERPRETATION
80–90%	Mild osteopenia
75–80%	Moderate osteopenia
75% or less	Osteoporosis

You should be aware that it is possible to have normal bone density in some spinal vertebrae and low bone density in others. But a low reading in *any* bone is a sign of increased risk.

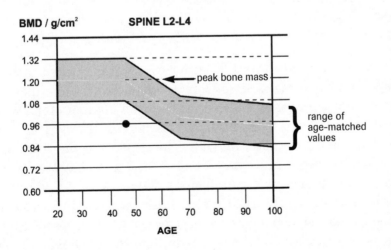

Medical Society, which should be able to tell you what equipment is being used in area medical groups, hospitals and research centers. You may also contact the National Osteoporosis Foundation, 1150 17th Street NW, Suite 500, Washington, DC 20036, which can provide a list of facilities in your area that perform bone density testing.

Are bone density tests worth the cost? Densitometry is not exactly cheap, and many insurance companies don't provide coverage for it. So you may be asking yourself whether it's worthwhile to have your bone density tested if you have to pay for it yourself.

The answer, in our opinion, is definitely yes. Let's say you pay $150 for a DEXA test. If you find out that your bone mass is high, you won't need preventive therapy (average cost of hormones: $20 per month). Over the years you will save thousands of dollars. If, on the other hand, you find out your bone mass is dangerously low, the cost of the test is minor compared to what can happen if your spine collapses or you break a hip.

If you can't afford a bone density test of the hip or spine, you could consider having the less expensive radiographic densitometry test. Or, you might be able to take part in a research study, especially if you live near an academic medical center. For information, contact the department that treats osteoporosis or metabolic bone diseases. Of course, no test will be effective, or cost effective, if you don't follow the recommendations for preventing bone loss.

National implications: Health care costs associated with osteoporotic fractures in 1995 were estimated at $13.8 billion. As the population ages, it is expected that the number of individuals in the age range of highest risk will increase dramatically; the incidence of hip fractures in the U.S. may triple by the year 2040.

At least two studies have found that bone density testing can reduce health care costs by millions of dollars. A 1992 study by the National Institutes of Health estimates that screening with bone density tests and then treating osteopenic women with hormone therapy could save an estimated $27.6 million over the next 40 years.

A more recent study conducted by the National Osteoporosis

Foundation (NOF) is far more optimistic. The NOF estimates that Medicare coverage of bone density testing for selected women ages 65 to 69 would cost $5.6 to $11.2 million per year. After about 5 years, the savings would total $233 to $466 million per year! Additional savings would come from fewer nursing home stays, fewer physician visits and enhanced earnings of the patient.

LAB TESTS FOR DETECTING BONE LOSS

If you already have bone loss, there are laboratory tests that go hand-in-hand with bone density testing to provide additional information. You can find out how fast you are losing bone (especially important when you are undergoing treatment), whether new bone is being formed, and whether bone loss is caused by osteoporosis or by another bone disorder.

If a bone density test shows you have been losing bone mass, your doctor may order one or more of the following tests.

Urine tests

Since food can affect the levels of calcium and other compounds in your urine, these tests are performed on the second voided sample of urine in the morning after an overnight fast.

Calcium-to-creatinine ratio: Creatinine is a breakdown product of metabolism; when measured in the urine as a ratio with the amount of calcium in the same urine sample, it reflects the amount of calcium being lost from the bones. Ratios over 0.16 indicate that, for some reason, bone loss has been accelerated.

Urinary collagen and bone collagen cross-links: In bone, collagen fibrils are joined together by linking bridges (peptides) called "cross-links." After the collagen is absorbed, the cross-links are excreted in the urine. The excretion of urinary collagen cross-links has been shown to be the most sensitive and specific marker of bone resorption (breakdown).

Collagen cross-link excretion significantly increases after menopause and is returned to premenopausal levels with hormone therapy or other effective antiresorptive therapy.

Two new tests in this category can help predict accelerated bone loss with great accuracy. *Pyrilinks D* involves measuring a substance found in bone and cartilage called deoxypyridinoline (D-PYR). *Osteomark* monitors bone loss by assessing the urinary excretion of another collagen cross-link, called n-telopeptide (N-Tx), which comes exclusively from bone.

Blood tests

Tests for calcium, phosphorus, and alkaline phosphatase (an enzyme involved in calcium metabolism) are the most common blood tests.

An abnormal level of calcium or phosphorus usually indicates a secondary cause of excessive bone loss, such as overactivity of the parathyroid or thyroid gland. This should be performed at least once as a baseline, and then repeated according to your needs as assessed by your physician.

To ensure that the estrogen you take is being absorbed, your physician can monitor blood estrogen levels (estradiol) or test your blood for levels of follicle stimulating hormone (FSH). The latter should decrease as blood estrogen values increase.

If your bone density is not responding to ERT, a bone specific alkaline phosphatase test to monitor your bone remodeling cycle should be considered. *Ostase* is a test that measures the blood level of bone specific alkaline phosphatase, which can help determine whether new bone is being formed. It is most useful in monitoring the effectiveness of treatment in women who have hyperparathyroidism or are taking sodium fluoride. Abnormal levels of alkaline phosphatase may indicate osteomalacia, the bone loss condition linked with vitamin D deficiency.

Other blood tests can be performed if you have symptoms in addition to low bone mass, or if hormone or other therapy doesn't stop loss of bone mass. Your physician may look for a secondary cause of osteoporosis—perhaps from an underlying medical condition that must be treated to prevent further bone loss, or from medication that will need to be adjusted or changed.

6 How Nutrition Can Help Prevent Bone Loss

O verall good nutrition is essential for the health of your bones. Calcium and vitamin D are particularly crucial. This is true at any age. It is true whether or not you exercise regularly. It is true whether or not you are are taking hormones or other bone-conserving drugs.

THE IMPORTANCE OF CALCIUM

Calcium is a major component of bone—bone is roughly two-thirds mineral by weight, and calcium makes up about 40% of that mineral. So it is certainly reasonable to assume that a diet low in calcium would compromise bone health.

Over the years, calcium's role in maintaining bone health has been controversial and confusing. When osteoporosis first started making headlines in the early 1980s, calcium was touted in news reports as the cure-all. Then came word that calcium didn't prevent fractures or slow bone loss in postmenopausal women as effectively as estrogen.

Even recent studies have been maddeningly inconsistent. Robert P. Heaney, MD, one of the country's leading experts on calcium and bones, reviewed 43 studies published between 1988 and 1993: 26 of them reported that calcium intake was associated with an increase in bone mass (or a decrease in bone loss or fractures), and 16 did not.

Though the research hasn't been consistent, the vast majority of studies to date show a relationship between calcium consumption and bone health. There is convincing evidence that adequate calcium intake is essential throughout life.

Laboratory animals fed a diet deficient in calcium develop osteoporosis.

In a classic study from Yugoslavia, researchers compared bone mass in two groups: the average daily calcium intake of one group (940 mg) was twice that of the other (441 mg). Women in the high-calcium group had stronger bones at skeletal maturity and a lower incidence of hip fractures later in life than those in the low-calcium group.

American women with osteoporosis typically consume less calcium than non-osteoporotic women and, in addition, they absorb it less efficiently from the foods they eat. Studies of British women corroborate these findings.

A recent review of the studies evaluating the efficacy of exercise to increase bone mass concluded that a daily intake of at least 1,000 mg of calcium is required to produce a bone building result.

Tufts University researchers recently reported that adding 500 mg of calcium and 700 IU of vitamin D to the diets of 176 men and 213 women over age 65 for three years significantly reduced their risk of non-vertebral fractures.

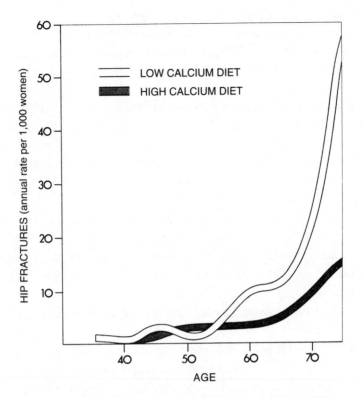

**INCIDENCE OF HIP FRACTURES RELATED TO AGE
AND DIETARY CALCIUM IN YUGOSLAVIAN WOMEN**

A systematic review of the literature and a definitive study published in the New England Journal of Medicine both confirm that dietary calcium and/or calcium supplements do reduce bone loss and osteoporotic fractures in people over 65 years of age.

Here's something to else to consider: Even if calcium did not have a part in building bone, too little calcium in your diet would result in a loss of bone mass. There must be enough calcium in your bloodstream for heart function, muscle contraction, blood pressure regulation and other important functions. If the calcium isn't there, it is taken from the bones. You need enough dietary calcium to prevent that.

HOW MUCH CALCIUM DO YOU NEED?

To find out if your daily calcium intake is sufficient, take a few minutes to fill out our Calcium Questionnaire on pages 221 and 222.

Your body needs calcium for bone mineralization, and adequate calcium intake is important throughout your life. Yet at almost every age from puberty through the postmenopausal years, most American women don't get enough calcium in their diet. On any given day, one-quarter of them will consume less than 300 milligrams of calcium.

At every age the needs are different. As people get older, their bodies become less efficient in handling dietary calcium. This is due, at least in part, to a gradual decline in the body's capacity to metabolize vitamin D into its active form (necessary for calcium absorption).

Children may absorb up to 75% during periods of rapid skeletal growth, adults only 30 to 50%, menopausal women even less. A study by Dr. Heaney reported an additional 9% decline after menopause, and he estimates that a woman can expect a 20% to 25% decline from ages 40 to 60. This decline is even greater after age 70 and in women who have osteoporosis. Impaired stomach acid production in many elderly women further limits calcium absorption.

This age-related reduction in absorption is one reason women need so much calcium and may help explain why we all lose some bone as we grow older.

In the teens   Just when a teenage girl's calcium requirement goes up to 1,600 milligrams, her calcium intake is likely to go down. Poor dietary habits—soda pop **Over half of all girls under age 15 do not get enough calcium.** instead of milk, potato chips instead of vegetables, for example—are a major source of the problem. Chronic dieting is another. By age 15, more than half of American girls have a daily calcium intake below the Recommended Dietary Allowance (RDA).

In a study of 48 healthy girls ages 9-13 years, half had their diet supplemented with dairy products that brought their daily calcium intake up to 1,200 mg, while the others ate their usual diet. The higher calcium group achieved greater bone density than the control subjects.

Pennsylvania State University researchers added 500 mg of calcium citrate maleate to the diets of 12- and 14-year old girls and found that after 4 years, their skeletal mass increased by 4%. If that level of improvement could be sustained until their bones were fully matured, it would translate to as much as a 50% reduction in the risk of fractures from osteoporosis.

In an Indiana University study of identical twins ages 6 to 14, the twin given a calcium supplement in addition to a diet adequate in calcium had higher bone mass after three years than her sister who didn't receive a supplement.

In young adulthood   As women grow older, the problem gets worse. More than two-thirds of women in the 18-to-30 age range consume less than the RDA for calcium. After age 35, three out of four women have a calcium intake below the RDA.

RECOMMENDED CALCIUM AND VITAMIN D

AGE AND LIFE-STAGE	CALCIUM (mg)	VITAMIN D (IU)
Children (ages 4–8)	800–1,000	200
Pre-adolescents and adolescents (9–18)	1,300	200
Women (to 31, with functioning ovaries)	1,000–1,200	200
Pregnant/lactating women over 20	1,000–1,100	200
Perimenopausal (32–50, functioning ovaries)	1,000–1,200	400
Postmenopausal women on therapy*	1,000–1,400	600
Postmenopausal women not on therapy*	1,400–2,000	600–800

* natural or surgical menopause

Recommendations are based on best current information in published clinical resources and accepted medical practice, and incorporate the 1997 federal guidelines from the National Academy of Sciences.

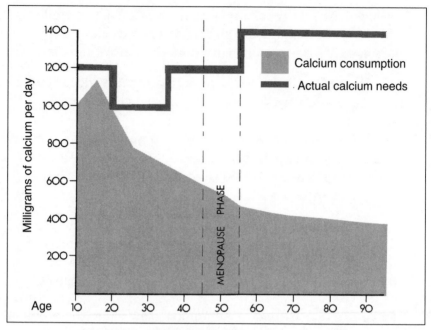

WOMEN'S CALCIUM NEEDS AND INTAKE WITH AGE

In the middle years and beyond The average American woman over 45 consumes very little calcium: only 450 to 650 milligrams each day. This is compounded by physical changes associated with aging.

> Tufts University researchers demonstrated that postmenopausal women with dietary calcium below 400 mg a day had a slowdown in bone loss when they took a 500 mg calcium supplement.

> In a New Zealand study, postmenopausal women whose calcium intake was about 750 mg/day had a slowdown in bone loss when they took a 1,000-mg supplement.

HOW TO STAY IN CALCIUM BALANCE

Calcium balance is the net of the processes through which calcium enters and leaves the body. If you take in and absorb more calcium than you lose (through sweat, urine, or feces), then you are in *positive calcium balance.* Losing more than you take in puts you in *negative calcium balance.*

If you stay in negative calcium balance for very long, your body leaches calcium from your skeleton to make up for its losses. It has been estimated that 25 years of a negative balance can result in your losing up to one-third of your skeletal bone mass.

25 years of negative calcium balance can cause you to lose 1/3 of your bone mass.

How much calcium your body absorbs and how much it excretes is affected not only by your daily calcium intake but by a number of other factors, both dietary and nondietary. Here are some ways to help stay in calcium balance.

Maintain a calcium-rich diet By far the most important way to stay in calcium balance is to make a conscious effort to consume enough of the mineral on a regular basis. The following are all especially good sources of calcium.

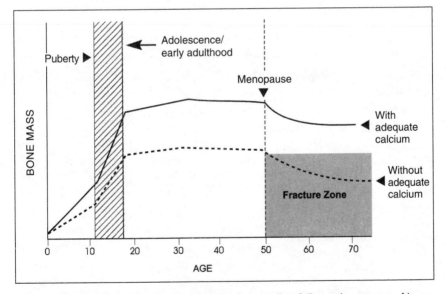

BONE MASS IN RELATION TO CALCIUM. The upper line follows the course of bone mass accrual and loss in a group of women who maintain adequate calcium intake. The lower line indicates women without adequate calcium intake. Each group maintains an appropriate lifestyle (exercise, etc.). Note the differences during puberty, when adequate calcium can help prevent fractures later in life.

Dairy products. Milk is the ideal calcium source and the one most women rely on. Not only does it contain about 300 milligrams of calcium in every cup, it is fortified with vitamin D to ensure absorption of the calcium. Milk also contains lactose, a sugar that aids in calcium absorption.

Yogurt has even more calcium than milk: 415 milligrams in an 8-ounce serving. You can also drain off the whey from yogurt (easy with a commercial filter such as Mike's Famous Yogurt Cheese Maker) to make yogurt cheese, a high-calcium, low calorie substitute for cream cheese or sour cream. Cheese is another excellent source.

Milk and yogurt come in low-fat and non-fat forms. Yogurt cheese adds variety to your meals.

Hard cheeses (such as Swiss or cheddar) contain much more calcium than soft cheeses (brie, for example). Milk and other dairy products are readily available in low-fat and non-fat varieties, so you do not need to be concerned with dietary fat.

What if you don't eat dairy products? Although dairy products are the principal source of calcium in our culture, this is not the case everywhere around the globe. The Chinese, for instance, depend on soybean products and leafy green vegetables.

Leafy green vegetables and broccoli. Broccoli and many leafy green vegetables, such as kale, turnip greens, collard greens, mustard greens and Swiss chard, are full of calcium and other valuable vitamins and minerals. (One exception is raw spinach, whose calcium is bound by oxalates and is poorly absorbed by the body.) One cup of collards provides 15% of the U.S. RDA for calcium and only 27 calories. Scotch kale has 17% calcium and 37 calories.

Tofu. When coagulated with *calcium sulfate*, tofu is an excellent source of calcium. This mild, no-cholesterol food is made by pressing the curds of soybean milk into blocks. A single 4-ounce serving contains about 150 milligrams of calcium. Tofu is also a good source of iron, potassium, the essential B vitamins and vitamin E.

Tofu coagulated with calcium sulfate is an excellent source of calcium.

Described as a "culinary chameleon," tofu takes on the flavors of whatever it is cooked with. It can be eaten plain without cooking, or used as an ingredient in soups, stews, salads, vegetable or egg dishes, or desserts.

Always buy the freshest tofu you can find. And be sure to check the label for calcium sulfate; the calcium content of tofu made with other coagulants is considerably lower.

Canned fish. Canned salmon and sardines are high in calcium as long as you include the bones (virtually all of the calcium is in the bones), which are soft enough to eat.

Water. There is calcium in your water, too! If you live in an area with "soft" water, you can get 10 to 30 milligrams of calcium per quart of tap water. If you have "hard" water, a quart will contain up to 100 milligrams.

Eat calcium-fortified foods These products can be a real boon. Calcimilk, for example, contains 500 mg of calcium per 8-ounce glass, roughly 200 mg more than regular milk. (It also has reduced lactose, making it easier for the lactose-intolerant to digest.) An 8-ounce glass of calcium-fortified orange juice provides 293 mg of calcium (Minute Maid) or 333 mg (Tropicana). You can even get calcium-fortified bread (Wonder Bread, 580 mg in 2 slices).

HIGH CALCIUM FOODS		
FOOD	QTY	CALCIUM (mg)*
Milk	1 cup	300
Cheddar cheese	1 oz	200
Swiss cheese	1 oz	275
Yogurt (plain)	1 cup	415
Yogurt cheese	1 cup	560
Beet greens	1 cup	100
Broccoli, cooked	1 cup	100
Collards, cooked	1 cup	350
Dandelion greens	1 cup	140
Kale, cooked, chopped	1 cup	180
Mustard or turnip greens, cooked	1 cup	190
Spinach, cooked	1 cup	100
Swiss chard	1 cup	75
Salmon, canned, with bones	3 oz	200
Sardines, with bones	4	180
Tofu (make with calcium carbonate)	4 oz	150

* approximate

TIPS TO ENHANCE THE CALCIUM IN YOUR MEALS

1. Make your own soup. Add a little vinegar when preparing stock from bones; the vinegar will dissolve the calcium out of the bones, making one pint of soup equal in calcium to a quart or more of milk. Add more calcium with tofu, cubes of cheese, dark green leafy vegetables or powdered nonfat milk.

2. Before cooking meat that contains bone, use vinegar to tenderize the meat (the vinegar taste will disappear). The juice that remains after cooking contains dissolved calcium, so use it in gravy, soup stock, etc.

3. Substitute shredded or grated cheese for butter on vegetables.

4. Make salads from the deep green lettuce leaves, which are richer in calcium than the paler leaves. Toss with tofu cubes, shredded cheese, nuts, sardines or salmon (with bones).

5. Garnish *everything* with cubes of cheese or tofu.

6. For pickling fruits or vegetables, use calcium chloride instead of sodium chloride (table salt).

7. Add powdered nonfat dry milk to everything you can. It makes skim milk, coffee and tea "thicker" and creamier, and enhances the flavor of cream soups and casseroles.

8. When baking bread, cake, cookies or muffins, add about 1/4 cup powdered nonfat milk to the recipe.

Calcium fortified products may cost more than the regular versions. You will have to judge for yourself whether their convenience is worth the additional cost.

Take a calcium supplement Increasing your calcium intake with food should be your first priority, since food also supplies other nutrients you need to keep healthy. But sometimes it's hard to get all the calcium you need from diet alone. Calcium supplements are an easy way to bridge the gap between dietary calcium and the amount recommended to protect your bones.

Is the calcium just as good as that in food? Several studies have shown that it is. In fact, the calcium in some types of supplements may be absorbed even better than calcium in food.

But remember, too much of almost *any* supplement can lead to nutritional imbalances, and calcium is no exception. (Large doses of calcium can interfere with iron absorption, for example.)

What about lead contamination? Tablets made from bone meal once contained a high amount of lead. Manufacturers have since removed most of the lead, so this is no longer a health risk. Still, all calcium supplements can contain traces of lead, since calcium salts come from natural sources, and lead is found naturally in the environment. The amount in calcium pills is negligible and does not pose a health threat when they are used in moderation.

Which calcium supplement is best? There is an overwhelming variety of products available in tablet, powder and liquid forms. Some are combined with vitamin D to aid in absorption, some are combined with magnesium and other minerals, and some come in multivitamin form. (Magnesium competes with calcium in the body and needs to be balanced with your overall calcium intake.)

Different types of supplements provide different amounts of *elemental* calcium—actual *pure* calcium, which is what the government recommendations are based on. But some brands use "500 mg of calcium" to mean 500 mg of *total* calcium and others mean 500 mg of *elemental* calcium. It makes a big difference! If a 500-mg tablet provides 500 milligrams of *total* calcium, you would not take 2 tablets to meet a goal of 1,000 mg; you would need 5 tablets, since each one contains only 200 mg of elemental calcium.

ELEMENTAL CALCIUM IN COMMON SUPPLEMENTS

FORM OF CALCIUM	IF TOTAL CALCIUM IN 1 TABLET IS	ELEMENTAL CALCIUM IN THAT TABLET IS	IT TAKES THIS MANY TABLETS FOR 1,000 MG CALCIUM
Calcium carbonate	500 mg	200 mg	5
Tribasic calcium phosphate	800 mg	304 mg	4
Calcium citrate	950 mg	200 mg	5
Calcium lactate	650 mg	84 mg	12
Calcium gluconate	500 mg	45 mg	22

Get in the habit of reading labels to find out how much elemental calcium is in each tablet. If that

The fewer tablets you have to take, the more likely you will take them.

information is not on the label, ask the pharmacist. Or look for a toll-free phone number on the label to call for information.

These are the most widely-used types of calcium supplements:

Calcium carbonate (Caltrate, Os-Cal, Tums) is usually the least expensive and supplies the highest amount of calcium per tablet. It is readily absorbed by most women, but is absorbed less well than calcium citrate by women with impaired stomach acid production—a common condition among postmenopausal and elderly women. Taking a supplement with food usually solves the problem.

Tribasic calcium phosphate (Posture) has not been as thoroughly tested as other forms of calcium. Some laboratory studies have suggested that it may be less soluble than other forms and therefore not as readily available to the body. However, a French study involving some 3,200 women found that it substantially reduced both bone loss and fractures in women who took it.

Calcium citrate (Citracal) is one of the fastest to dissolve and best absorbed, especially when taken on an empty stomach. But based on the amount of elemental calcium, you will need to take more tablets than calcium carbonate or tribasic calcium phosphate.

Calcium lactate dissolves more reliably than calcium carbonate, but it has less elemental calcium, so you will have to take more tablets.

Calcium gluconate (Kalcinate) is more soluble than calcium carbonate but contains only a small amount of elemental calcium (10 mg for every 1,000 mg of total calcium).

Calcium levulinate has a low percentage of elemental calcium (130 mg per 1,000 mg of total calcium) and has a bitter, salty taste.

Bone meal and *dolomite* are high in calcium: 1 teaspoon of bone meal contains 120 mg; 1 teaspoon of dolomite contains 1,180 mg.

Calcium chloride is good for pickling but it is not a good supplement because it tends to irritate the stomach.

Chelated calcium is said to improve absorption, but there is no evidence that it is better absorbed than nonchelated supplements.

WHO MAY NEED A CALCIUM SUPPLEMENT?

The following women have increased calcium needs. If you find yourself on this list and are not getting enough calcium from your diet, you should consider a supplement.

• *Perimenopausal women* (ages 45–55). Hormonal changes preceding and following menopause make it harder to stay in calcium balance.

• *Estrogen-deprived women* (naturally or surgically menopausal, not on therapy). Not only does their low estrogen level make them prone to rapid bone loss, they absorb calcium less efficiently.

• *Women of all ages who exercise regularly.* Exercise increases bone matrix (soft new bone tissue), which requires adequate calcium for mineralization. The more regularly and strenuously they exercise, the greater is their need for calcium.

• *Women who have a high intake of protein, fiber, sodium or caffeine, or use antacids with aluminum;* these cause the body to excrete calcium.

• *Women who have had recent illness, injury or major surgery.* Bed rest and reduced activity makes them prone to rapid bone loss.

• *Women who have a chronically low calcium intake,* as from a strict vegetarian diet, lactose-intolerance, chronic dieting or eating disorders.

• *Women on a therapeutic low-sodium diet (usually with high blood pressure).* Many calcium-rich dairy products are also high in sodium.

Can you have too much calcium?   Yes, but it's not easy. For most adults, more than 2,500 milligrams is the safe upper limit, according to the 1997 guidelines from the National Academy of Sciences. Most adult women only take in 450 mg of calcium per day from dietary sources. It is almost impossible to exceed the upper limit of calcium intake through diet alone.

Many people are afraid that "excess" milk consumption will lead to kidney stones. The fact is, women rarely get kidney stones.

When they do, it is usually because they lack certain enzymes needed to keep calcium and urine in solution, and not because of high calcium intake.

A recent study led by Gary C. Curhan, MD, at Harvard School of Public Health followed over 45,000 men who had no recent history of kidney stones. Researchers found that those with high calcium diets (1,300 mg) cut their risk of developing kidney stones in half, compared to those with the least calcium (500 mg).

This finding should apply equally to women. Actually, it is women who have too little calcium and have a diet high in oxalates who may increase their risk of developing kidney stones. Still, if you have a history of kidney stones, consult your physician before taking a calcium supplement.

HOW TO GET THE MOST FROM CALCIUM SUPPLEMENTS

1. Take the supplement at bedtime. The body loses larger amounts of calcium when you sleep.

2. Take no more than 500 mg at a time. Calcium is best absorbed in small amounts, so if your daily dosage exceeds 500 mg, take 500 mg at bedtime, 500 mg in the morning, and any additional to make up your daily requirement at midday.

3. Take supplements with a little food, orange juice, milk or yogurt. The acid in the orange juice and the lactose in milk and yogurt help increase absorption.

4. If you also take an iron supplement, take it at a different time of day. Iron interferes with calcium absorption.

5. Test your supplement. Some of them don't break up in your stomach as readily as others. Place the tablet in a glass with a few ounces of room-temperature white vinegar and stir vigorously every 5 minutes or so. At least 75% of the tablet should disintegrate within 30 minutes.

GET ENOUGH VITAMIN D

Activated vitamin D, the "sunshine vitamin," is vital for the creation of new bone—calcium absorption and bone mineralization cannot take place without it. Some experts believe that a deficiency of vitamin D in itself causes osteoporosis and is more common than people realize. (About one-third of hip fracture patients are deficient in vitamin D.) Like osteoporosis, vitamin D deficiency has no symptoms.

Vitamin D deficiency can cause osteoporosis.

The recommended dietary allowance for women over 30 is 400 IU (international units). As you get older, it takes even more to satisfy your body's requirements. Women over age 50 need 600 to 800 IU of vitamin D per day.

Over 30, you need 400 IU of vitamin D per day. Over 50, you may need 800 IU per day.

In a study at Tufts University, women given 700 IU of vitamin D lost less bone than those who took 100 IU a day.

Vitamin D from the sun. Although the sun is a good source of this vitamin, you can't count on it. One reason is that you never know how much you are getting—it is impossible to measure how much sunshine produces a certain amount of vitamin D. The amount depends on the sun's intensity, your length of time in the sun, plus atmospheric conditions and other variables, such as time of day, season of year, where you live (at higher latitudes the winter sun can't make vitamin D), your skin pigmentation, etc.

In another Tufts University study, a group of post-menopausal women became vitamin D-deficient during the winter months, when exposure to sunlight was limited. When spring came, those whose vitamin D from food and supplements was below 220 IU daily had higher levels of bone-dissolving parathyroid hormone in their blood.

Women in Maine lost about 3% of bone mass during the winter, related to a decrease in vitamin D levels. Part of the loss was recovered during the summer.

In a study we conducted, women living in Florida had two times the level of vitamin D as women living in Finland.

Use of a sunscreen can also interfere with the beneficial effects of the sun; a sunscreen blocks the ultraviolet B rays that trigger the skin's manufacture of vitamin D. For the same reason, sun coming through the window is of no value.

At least one preliminary study has shown that women who used a sunscreen at midday in summer, when vitamin D levels are at their peak, had a 50% lower blood level of vitamin D than those who did not use a sunscreen.

Some experts estimate that a fair-skinned woman can meet her vitamin D requirement from daily sun exposure of 15 minutes to 1 hour (without a sunscreen). Of course, your vitamin D requirement should be balanced with the need to protect your skin from excessive sun exposure.

Vitamin D from food. Vitamin D in the diet is fairly limited, with small amounts in fatty fish (sardines, salmon, herring, mackeral, swordfish), butter, egg yolks, organ meats such as liver, and cod liver oil. Milk that has been fortified with vitamin D is a good source, but part of the problem is that most women don't drink milk. If your doctor has any concern that you may be vitamin D-deficient, it can be measured with a blood test. Two forms are detectable: 25-hydroxyvitamin D, formed in the liver, and the fully active form, 1,25-dihydroxyvitamin D, which is converted to the active form by the kidney.

What you can do. If you are under age 50 and a regular milk drinker who gets some sun exposure on a daily basis, you will likely meet the RDA of 400 IU (international units).

If you are over 50, you should definitely consider taking a supplement to meet your increased need of 600 to 800 IU per day. It's best not to rely on food sources because **Too much vitamin D can actually stimulate bone loss.** even those that supply vitamin D have very little of it. No need to become overzealous, though: too much vitamin D can actually stimulate bone loss. You should take no more than 1,000 IU per day, not counting exposure to sunlight (the body destroys any excess that comes from sunlight).

GET ENOUGH VITAMIN K

Vitamin K is a fat-soluble vitamin that plays an important role in bone mineralization, and there's some evidence that a deficiency may be instrumental in the development of osteoporosis.

Bone GLA protein, a peptide produced by the bone-building osteoblasts, declines in vitamin K–deficient blood. Hip fracture patients have been found to have a low blood level of vitamin K. And vitamin K supplements have been found to reduce the amount of calcium excreted in urine of women with osteoporosis.

What you can do. Although more needs to be learned about the exact role of vitamin K in maintaining bone health, it certainly wouldn't hurt to ensure that you're getting enough in your diet. Fortunately, that isn't too hard to do. The RDA for women is 65 micrograms. You can get that from a balanced diet that regularly (4 or 5 times a week) includes leafy green vegetables, especially cabbage, broccoli, turnip greens and lettuce.

BEWARE OF THE "BONE ROBBERS"

Many substances can cause calcium to be excreted at a higher-than-normal rate, putting you at risk of a negative calcium balance. These include excessive amounts of protein, salt, caffeine, oxylates and phytates, fiber and vitamin A. Dieting and stress can cause you to excrete calcium, too. As long as you are aware of these "robbers," you can start protecting yourself from them.

Too much protein Protein is known to increase calcium excretion. The calcium loss from large amounts of protein is quick and dramatic, and resultant bone loss can easily double or triple.

Women with normal protein intake (average 65 grams per day) were given a 50% increase in protein. The result was that they lost an extra 26 mg of calcium per day. Translated into bone loss, this is about 1% of bone mass per year, which is similar to the bone loss that occurs after menopause.

It's true that you need a certain amount of protein to provide the nine essential amino acids that your body can't make by itself. Most Americans, however, consume far more than they need. Generally speaking, about 15% of your total daily calories should come from protein.

Red meat adds to the problem. In addition to being a high protein source, its acidity promotes the excretion of calcium into the urine. Red meat also contains a good deal of phosphorus, which may also predispose you to bone loss. A diet rich in meat is also high in fat, which is bad from the standpoint of cardiovascular health.

Red meat has more than one strike against it.

What you can do. One way to lower protein is to lower meat consumption. If you have meat daily, try cutting down to only a couple of times a week. Substitute vegetable proteins, tofu, fish or poultry for red meat proteins.

Are vegetarians better off? There's some evidence to suggest that vegetarian women have stronger, denser bones than women whose diets are heavy with meat; they appear to lose less bone and develop osteoporosis far less often than non-vegetarians.

In one study of women between the ages of 50 and 89, those who ate meat regularly were compared to lacto-ovo vegetarians (dairy products but no meat). Both groups had comparable amounts of calcium in their diets, yet the meat eaters lost 35% of their bone mass and the vegetarians lost only 18%.

In another study, the average bone density of vegetarians in their 70s was greater than that of the meat-eaters in their 50s!

But, in a study we conducted with Rogene Tesar, PhD, we found no differences in the vertebral bone densities of vegetarian and non-vegetarian women.

The apparent inconsistencies in the research may be due to the different kinds of vegetarian diets. The lack of animal protein protects bone, but this may be offset by the oxylates and phytates in many vegetables and grains. Strict vegetarians, also known as vegans—those who eliminate both meat *and* dairy products from their diet—will have a harder time staying in calcium balance and, in fact, may be at a greater risk of developing osteoporosis unless they take supplements.

Case history: Teresa, age 49

The dietary practices of some vegetarians can lead to osteopenia despite adequate hormone therapy.

Teresa's ovaries were removed when she was 37 years old. She began taking oral estrogen (Premarin,1.25 mg daily) to help protect against heart disease and osteoporosis. Twelve years later she came to the clinic because of vaginal dryness; she also wanted a second opinion as to whether she should continue taking estrogen to prevent osteoporosis.

During her evaluation, we learned that Teresa was a vegetarian who excluded all meat and dairy products from her diet. Her calcium intake was only 141 mg per day. She consumed virtually no vitamin D. Bone density testing of her 1st and 2nd lumbar vertebrae in the spine revealed that they were just 75% of peak bone mass. This indicated that she was at risk of fracturing one of these bones.

We recommended that Teresa continue her hormone therapy, and we emphasized the importance of supplementing her diet with at least 1,500 mg of calcium daily, along with a multivitamin. This, together with additional exercise, should improve her bone density over the next several years.

Too much sodium   Table salt is made of sodium chloride crystals. Sodium is an essential nutrient—our bodies require it for maintenance of blood volume, regulation of fluid balance, transport of molecules across cell walls, and transmission of impulses along nerve fibers.

But most of us eat too much sodium, and that is not healthy for a number of reasons. Besides raising blood pressure in salt-

FOODS WITH HIGH SODIUM CONTENT

OVER 1,000 MILLIGRAMS	AMOUNT	SODIUM (mg)
Ham, cured lean	6 oz (3 slices)	1,750
Corned beef	6 oz (4 slices)	1,600
Crabmeat, canned	1 can (4 oz)	1,250
Turkey sub, fast food	1	1,190
Beef broth, canned	1 cup	1,152
Steak fajita wrap, fast food	1	1,130
Soup, canned (chicken, chicken noodle, onion)	1 cup	1,100
Hamburger, fast food	1	1,070
Soy sauce	1 Tbsp	1,029
Grilled chicken salad, fast food	1 serving	1,020
Pretzels, regular twist	10 (1 oz)	1,010

500 TO 1,000 MILLIGRAMS		
Spaghetti with tomato sauce and cheese	1 cup	955
Tomato soup, canned	1 cup	872
Sauerkraut, canned	1/2 cup	777
Tomato juice, canned	6 fl oz	659
Frankfurter, all meat	1	639
Potatoes,mashed,milk & salt	1 cup	632
Cheese, parmesan, grated	1 oz	528
Cheese, cottage	1/2 cup	500

150 TO 500 MILLIGRAMS		
Beans, baked, canned	1/2 cup	464
Spinach, canned	1/2 cup	455
Cheese, American	1 slice (1 oz)	406
Corn flakes	1 oz (1 cup)	350
Bacon	4 slices (1 oz)	348
Corn, creamed, canned	1/2 cup	336
Tuna or sardines, canned	1 can (3 1/4 oz)	328
Beans, green, canned	1/2 cup	319
Roll, hard	1 roll	313
Asparagus, canned	4 spears	298
Potato chips	14 (1 oz)	285
Sausage, pork	1 patty (2 oz)	259
Buttermilk	8 fl oz	257
Peas, canned	1/2 cup	247
Pickle, dill	1 spear	232
Corn chips, regular	1 oz	231
French dressing	1 Tbsp	214
Catsup	1 Tbsp	156
Cashews, dry-roasted, salted	1 oz	150

sensitive individuals (increasing the risk of hypertension, heart and vascular diseases, and kidney disease), salt can cause large amounts of calcium to be lost in the urine.

The more sodium in your diet, the more you excrete—and the more sodium you excrete, the more calcium you lose. Our bodies strive to maintain a balance of sodium and calcium. Eat too much salt and your body leaches calcium from your bones to make up the difference.

> In 1995, Australian researchers followed 100 post-menopausal women for 2 years and discovered that those who ate the most sodium lost the most bone from their hips and ankles. Women with the highest losses ate more than 3,000 mg of sodium per day.

Scientists say we need only 500 mg a day of sodium to stay healthy. Health experts recommend a daily limit of 2,400 mg. Whether that amount is low enough to preserve bone is unclear. But most of us consume 10 to 20 times that much.

To make things more confusing, if you live in a warm climate or exercise vigorously, perspiration could cause you to excrete 100% of your dietary sodium needs and thus require a higher daily salt intake than women living in more temporate climates.

A problem many women face is that many calcium-rich foods are loaded with hidden sodium. If you are on a salt-restricted diet, chances are your calcium intake becomes restricted as well.

Many calcium-rich roods are loaded with sodium.

In younger people, salt does not always have a negative result because it helps reabsorption of calcium by the kidney. Here's how it works:

As large amounts of salt are lost in the urine, blood levels of calcium are lowered, triggering the release of parathyroid hormone, which, in an attempt to normalize blood calcium, increases vitamin D production, which stimulates calcium absorption.

Older individuals are less able to adapt to this protective mechanism and therefore need to be more cautious about overloading with salt.

What you can do. Ten percent of the sodium in our diet occurs naturally in food, 15% comes from the salt we add in cooking or at the table (1 teaspoon contains 2,325 mg of sodium), and a whopping 75% comes from processed food. A bowl of canned chicken noodle soup delivers a day's worth of salt, as do many fast-food meals.

To achieve a safe range of sodium, stay away from processed foods and fast foods. Throw away your salt shaker and use a salt substitute or herbs and spices in cooking.

Using 1,000 milligrams as your target amount of sodium, try to estimate whether your salt consumption is too high. If your estimated total is 2,000 mg, balance it with an *extra 1,000 mg of dietary calcium* (over the amount you normally need). If you think your sodium comes to 3,000 mg, add an extra 1,700 mg of calcium. Conversely, by reducing dietary sodium from 2,000 to 1,200 mg, your calcium requirement can be decreased by 125–200 mg.

Too much caffeine   The actual effects of caffeine on the bones has not been thoroughly studied. We do know, however, that the more coffee (or tea, cola, etc.) you drink, the more calcium you lose from your body. The Framingham Study reported an increased risk of hip fractures among people who had two or more caffeinated beverages per day. But it is believed that this negative effect can be offset by the addition of dietary calcium.

A recent study, however, in the American Journal of Clinical Nutrition, found that caffeine does not weaken bones, even in women who drink 5 or more cups of coffee a day.

What you can do. We don't think it is necessary for you to swear off all coffee, tea and cola drinks. But until there is more research, we believe it is safer to keep your caffeine intake as low as you can. And compensate for the caffeine you do have with extra calcium in your diet or by taking a calcium supplement.

Oxalates and phytates   *Oxalates* are compounds found in green vegetables such as asparagus, beet greens, spinach, sorrel, dandelion greens and rhubarb. In the intestine, they combine with calcium to form large, insoluble complexes that cannot be absorbed. *Phytates* are phosphorus-containing compounds found principally in the outer husks of cereal grains, especially oatmeal and bran.

They, too, interfere with calcium absorption by combining with calcium in the intestine.

What you can do. It is not necessary to eliminate the above foods from your diet in order to maintain calcium balance. You should know, however, that you cannot depend on them as sources of calcium. Try to avoid eating calcium-rich foods (or supplements) at the same time as foods containing oxalates or phytates.

Too much fiber Fiber is an important part of your diet. It improves intestinal function, helps promote regularity, lowers cholesterol levels in the blood, improves glucose tolerance and reduces the risk of colon cancer. Good sources of fiber include bran, whole-wheat bread, brown rice, and fresh fruits and vegetables.

The problem with fiber is that it can prevent calcium from being absorbed. It does this by (1) combining with the calcium in the intestine, and (2) increasing the rate at which food is passed through the intestinal tract. Fiber derived from cereal sources contains phytates, thus limiting even further the amount of calcium that is absorbed.

What you can do. Fiber is essential, so you don't want to eliminate it from your diet. Most major health organizations recommend

---

BIOAVAILABILITY OF CALCIUM

Absorption of calcium depends on the total calcium content of the food as well as the presence of other constituents that either improve or hinder calcium absorption. For example, plants that contain phytates and especially oxylates will significantly reduce calcium absorption by forming insoluble calcium salts.

Actual absorption of calcium from food varies from one person to another. One study showed an average 12% decrease in calcium absorption from milk when it was added to wheat bran cereal, and an average 6.4% decrease in calcium absorption from milk when it was combined with spinach. Conversely, calcium absorption increased from 3% to 11% when additional milk was added to the spinach.

that you limit your fiber intake to no more than 35 grams per day. As with the foods containing oxalates and phytates, do not depend on high-fiber foods as a source of calcium, and try to avoid eating calcium-rich foods (or supplements) at the same time as high-fiber foods. If you use calcium supplements, take them (with a little food or orange juice) either 1 hour before or 2 hours after a high-fiber meal, or at bedtime.

Too much vitamin A   Too much vitamin A can stimulate bone loss; you only need 4,000 IU (international units) each day. Daily intake of more than 5,000 IU may stimulate bone loss, according to the American Society for Bone and Mineral Research.

What you can do. Check your vitamin labels, and don't over-do vitamin A-rich foods: liver, carrots, sweet potatoes, apricots, squash, cantaloupe, broccoli and peaches.

Dieting   American women are notorious dieters. Fad diets and fasting may be good ways to lose weight quickly (and almost always temporarily), but they are also good ways to lose calcium from your bones. Most reducing diets are extremely low in calcium and, of course, if you are fasting you are not getting any calcium at all.

Since your body requires a certain amount of calcium in the blood to keep your muscles and brain functioning and your blood clotting system in balance, it takes what it needs from the bones.

> Scientists at the National Institute on Aging studied 3,686 women ages 67 and older and found that those who had lost 10% or more of their weight since the age of 50 were twice as likely to fracture a hip.

What you can do. Calcium supplements will enable you to meet your calcium needs while still sticking to your diet.

Phosphorus   Along with calcium, phosphorus is a major component of bone. It is also an essential mineral found in every cell of your body and involved in virtually every metabolic process.

According to some scientists, however, too much phosphorus may lead to bone loss.

Some studies have shown that only very large amounts of phosphorus will have an appreciable effect. Others (on animals) have demonstrated bone loss when the amount of phosphorus in the diet greatly exceeds the amount of calcium. This appears to be the case in humans, as well, as evidenced by the high rate of bone loss in the Arctic Eskimos of Canada and Alaska, whose diet consists almost exclusively of phosphorus-rich walrus and seal meat. Arctic Eskimos start losing bone at an earlier age and lose 15 to 20% more bone than people in the continental U.S.

Estimates of phosphorus-to-calcium in the average American diet range from twice as much to four times as much. That is probably because so many popular foods are high in phosphorus, and it is widely used in food additives and is therefore a major component of processed foods (including low-fat processed cheeses).

High-phosphorus foods include the following: bacon, bologna, beef, bread, canned foods, cereal, cola drinks, corn, fish, oatmeal, popcorn, pork, potatoes, potato chips, poultry, tuna.

What you can do. Until we know exactly what role the ratio of calcium-to-phosphorus plays in bone loss, it is probably a good idea to avoid excesses of foods that contain large amounts of phosphorus. And remember that when you do have a lot of phosphorus, try to balance it with extra calcium.

Magnesium   Magnesium and calcium have similar functions in the body; both are abundant in bone tissue and are important for muscle contraction and nerve impulse transmission. Because of their similar functions, they compete with each other, and an excess of either one may interfere with the body's use of the other.

For this reason, it is essential to balance your intake of these minerals. The best calcium-to-magnesium ratio is 2-to-1; that is, you should have roughly twice as much calcium as magnesium.

What you can do. If you consume 1,400 mg of calcium per day, you should balance it with about 700 mg of magnesium. Foods high in magnesium include nuts, legumes (dried peas, beans), cereal grains, dark green vegetables and seafood.

Stress   The last "bone robber" is not part of your diet, but does affect it. Stress decreases the absorption of calcium and increases the amount lost in the urine. It also stimulates production of adrenal hormones, which increase bone breakdown.

What you can do. Whenever you are experiencing emotional or physical stress, try to increase your calcium.

7 How Exercise Can Help Prevent Bone Loss

If you want to prevent osteoporosis, you had better stand up and start moving. Regular moderate exercise is an important component of bone health and is one of the few ways to actually *increase* your bone mass.

Scientists still don't have all the answers about the specific effects of exercise on bone. It is clear, however, that world-class athletes, who make a lifelong habit of exercising, have denser bones than inactive people. And total inactivity leads to severe bone loss; with bed rest, for example, bone is lost at the alarming rate of 4% per month.

Exercise should be an integral part of your daily routine for osteoporosis prevention.

HOW EXERCISE BUILDS BONE

Just as muscles that are exercised become bigger and stronger, bones, too, respond to stress by becoming bigger and stronger (hypertrophy). And like muscles, they weaken and shrink if they are not used (atrophy).

The beneficial effects of exercise are site-specific, varying according to the activity. Runners and cyclists, for example, tend to have denser bones in the legs and hips, and tennis players have denser bones in their playing arm. Exercise also increases blood flow to the bones, bringing in bone-building nutrients and creating small electrical potentials in bone tissue that stimulate the growth of new bone.

Also affected are the hormones that control bone remodeling, all shifting the balance toward new bone formation.

> In a six-week program at Pennsylvania State University, middle-aged women who exercised increased their estrogen levels.

> A study at Case Western Reserve University (Cleveland) showed higher blood levels of estrogen immediately after each exercise session; the more intense the workout, the higher the increase in estrogen.

> Middle-aged men who rode exercise bicycles had lower levels of the harmful adrenal hormones after exercising.

The beneficial effects of exercise affect other bones as well as the exercised bones.

> Australian researchers found that women who exercised to increase the strength of their biceps muscles (in the arms) also had an increase in spinal bone density.

Exercise recommendations in this chapter are based on normal bone mass. Before beginning any new exercise regimen, discuss the program with your health care provider to assure that it is appropriate to your personal situation.

CAN EXERCISE STOP, SLOW OR REVERSE BONE LOSS?

It is good to know that athletes have bigger bones and that exercise somehow helps make bones stronger. But the more important question is, can exercise help slow bone loss in postmenopausal women . . . or possibly reverse it? A majority of studies have found that it can.

For one year, a group of postmenopausal women (average age 53) participated in a program recommended by the President's Council on Physical Fitness. Three times a week they performed warm-up, circulatory and conditioning exercises for 1 hour. They did not change their diet. The result was significantly improved calcium balance and no signs of bone loss.

Sixteen women ages 55 to 67 participated in a program of walking, running and calisthenics for 1 hour twice a week. At the end of eight months, bone density of the spine increased by 3 to 5%. A comparison group of non-exercising women had a 2.7% decrease in spinal bone density.

At Washington University (St. Louis), postmenopausal women who exercised (walking, jogging, stair climbing) for 45 minutes to an hour 3 times a week increased their bone mass an impressive 5.2% during the first nine months of the program, while sedentary women in the study lost 1.2% of bone mass. (After 22 months, the exercisers' bone mass had increased by 6.1%, while the non-exercisers continued to lose bone.)

Other studies have shown that exercise alone is not enough.

To test the effects of exercise combined with other preventive measures, Richard Prince, MD, studied four groups of postmenopausal women: (1) exercise only, (2) exercise + calcium supplement (1,000 mg/day), (3) exercise + estrogen, (4) no exercise, no calcium or estrogen.

After two years he found that the women who did nothing to protect their bones lost the most bone mass:

2.7%. The exercise-only group fared almost the same: a loss of 2.6%. The exercise-plus-calcium group had a small 0.5% loss of bone mass. The exercise-plus-estrogen group actually *gained* an average of 2.7% of bone mass.

Columbia University researchers found that in a group of postmenopausal women exercising at about the same level of intensity, those with a higher calcium intake had higher bone density in the spine.

Epidemiologist Bonny Specker of the University of Cincinnati Medical Center reviewed 17 studies that looked at how exercise affects bone density. She found that exercise made bones measurably stronger only when calcium was above 1,000 mg per day and the person was moderately active.

Our own year-long study found that surgically menopausal women who took estrogen and participated in a muscle-strengthening program (Nautilus equipment) 3 times per week had an 8% increase in spinal bone density, while sedentary women who took estrogen simply maintained bone mass.

Is it ever too late to begin exercising? Exercise builds bone more readily in younger women, particularly those who have not yet reached peak bone mass. Nevertheless, even postmenopausal women may be able to build bone mass by exercising regularly. We found that the sooner after menopause you begin, the more beneficial the exercise.

In a three-year study by Robert Recker, MD, women in their early 20s who were fairly active had a 6%–8% gain in bone mass, compared with only a 1/4%–2% increase in less active or inactive women.

In our study, women who began exercising within 5 years of their menopause experienced a greater slowdown of bone loss than women who started later.

WHAT TYPE OF EXERCISE IS BEST?

The best exercises are those that work the muscles harder than they would work normally. Activities such as weight lifting, walking, dancing, stair climbing, step aerobics, jogging, hiking and tennis are all effective at building bone.

Muscle strengthening exercises   Study after study has shown that weight training may be the best exercise for increasing bone density. The increase is directly proportional to the amount of stress applied.

Gail Dalsky and colleagues at Washington University reported impressive gains in spinal bone density with a combination aerobic and strength training program.

L. A. Pruitt and coworkers found that nine months of strength training in 13 recently postmenopausal women improved bone density in the spine by 1.6%, while a sedentary group had a loss of 3.6%.

A preliminary study at our clinic found that after 15 months, postmenopausal women participating in muscle strengthening exercises on Nautilus equipment achieved the same improvement in bone density as women taking hormone therapy.

In a Tufts University study, women who engaged in muscle-strengthening exercises had a 1% gain in bone density at the hip and spine, compared to a 2.5% loss at these sites in a control group who did not exercise.

Thirty-nine sedentary women, aged 50 to 70, were divided into two groups: for one year, half worked out on weight machines twice a week, 45 minutes per session; half remained sedentary. The women who exercised had better balance, stronger bones and more muscle than those who didn't exercise.

What you can do. We believe that the safest and most effective way to increase muscle strength is with variable resistance weight machines (such as Medex, Nautilus or Cybex). Most fitness centers and YMCAs have this equiment and a trained staff to teach you how to use it. Before you begin, a supervisor will establish your *repetition maximum* (the maximum weight you can lift at one time). Start with weights that are 50% of your repetition maximum and increase the weights by 10% every 2 weeks.

Before each exercise session, warm up with a few stretches. You may also want to increase your heart rate by walking or jogging in place for a few minutes. We recommend two sets of 8–12 repetitions, separated by a 1-minute rest period, for each of the large muscle groups: quadriceps, hamstrings, abdominals, and back muscles. *If you are at high risk for osteoporosis you should not do typical abdominal strengthening because it causes too much flexion force on the spinal column. Lumbar stabilization is better and safer.*

For the first month or two, try to plan 4 sessions a week of muscle-strengthening exercises to keep your muscles conditioned and help protect your bones. Thereafter, 3 sessions per week will suffice.

Free weights, such as barbells and dumbells, may be convenient because you can use them at home, **Free weights can increase your risk of injury, especially if your bone mass is low.** but they can increase the risk of injury. *Free weights should never be used by women who have osteopenia or osteoporosis without strict supervision and instruction.*

Walking Walking regularly is highly recommended; it is weightbearing and is not likely to harm the bony structure. But to be of value, it must be done properly.

Many people walk with the pelvis tilted forward and the head and shoulders out in front of the hips *(left figure, opposite page)*, causing the weight-bearing forces to fall in front of the hip and knee. This can cause hip, knee and back pain and lessen the effectiveness of the walking.

To obtain the maximum benefit you must walk with good body alignment: it is important for the weight-bearing forces to go through the hip joint *(right figure)*. To maximize weight-bearing through the legs, hip joints and thus throughout the body, bring the hips forward under the shoulders.

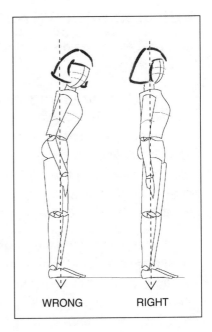

WRONG   RIGHT

You may feel a pulling or stretching sensation along the front of your hips and/or thighs; if so, it is not cause for concern— it just means that these areas need to be stretched out. If bringing the hips forward is very difficult for you, you may need to see a physical therapist to be evaluated for muscle tightness, which can be corrected with specific stretching and treatment.

Do *not* attempt to bring your shoulders back to correct your posture. It does not work and actually can cause more severe postural problems.

For best results, walking must be done regularly. Start out by making a commitment to yourself that you will stick with a program for 4–6 weeks. Begin by walking at whatever pace and distance your body will tolerate. Gradually work up to 30 to 45 minutes of brisk walking at least 4 times a week.

In a study of women between ages 41 and 70, Dr. Elizabeth Krall from Tufts University found that those who did 30 minutes of brisk walking a day slowed their rate of bone loss dramatically.

You don't have to walk for 30 minutes at a time, according to Dr. Krall: ten minutes here, 10 minutes there is fine—but you have to walk for at least 10 minutes at any one time to benefit.

WHICH EXERCISES ARE RIGHT FOR YOU?

Your best exercises depend on your age and also on your present bone density.

Children and young adults   This is the period of achieving peak bone mass. It's best to start exercise early in life, when your bones are still building density. Maintaining a healthy, active lifestyle at this stage is vital to future health. Do high impact activities such as ballet, gymnastics, soccer, volleyball, weight-training and basketball. But do not overexercise; warning signs include irregular periods or cessation of menses.

Mature adults   Your goal at this stage is to maintain as much bone mass and muscle strength as possible. Do vigorous low to moderate impact activities such as walking, jogging, running, aerobics, step aerobics, hiking, weight-training, rope skipping and cross-country skiing.

Menopausal and post-menopausal women   If a bone density test determines that your bone mass is normal, continue the exercise regimen you started in earlier adult years.

Since loss of estrogen after menopause accelerates bone loss, your exercise needs to combine movement, pull and stress on the long bones of the body. Walking, jogging, bicycling, hiking and rowing are all excellent load-bearing activities. "Load-bearing" refers to any exercise that forces your body to bear weight, even its own weight.

Women with osteopenia or osteoporosis   If a bone density test shows that you have started to lose bone, you will need to be more careful, both in your choice of activity and in how vigorously you exercise. For example, you should avoid flexion (forward bending) movements, which can increase your risk of fracture.

If your bone mass is low, opt for low to moderate impact activities such as walking, dancing, cross-country skiing, and supervised weight training. Site-specific exercise is also important to help build bone mass in your back and to reduce compression on the vertebral column.

The exercises in Chapter 10 are part of a program designed to treat osteoporosis, but they can also help prevent it. If you have osteoporosis and/or have sustained one or more fractures, these exercises will do no harm.

In addition, it would be a good idea to consult a physical therapist who specializes in the treatment of osteoporosis, to get help for any specific problems.

HOW MUCH EXERCISE DO YOU NEED?

We can't answer with certainty how much exercise is optimal for skeletal fitness. Our best recommendation is to exercise to achieve *cardiovascular fitness* and to improve your *muscle strength* and *endurance*. This way, you will be meeting two of the primary objectives of exercise in addition to helping to prevent bone loss.

You will also be controlling your weight, maintaining your flexibility, improving your balance, toning your muscles and reducing your risk of falling.

> We studied two groups of menopausal women who exercised on a treadmill 3 times a week. At the end of one year, their bone density was compared with a group who did not exercise. The non-exercisers lost bone mass. Those who exercised for 30 minutes lost bone mass at a slower rate. Those who exercised for 45 minutes had a slight increase in bone mass.

Very strenuous and prolonged physical training, on the other hand, can actually have a negative effect. Numerous studies have confirmed that female athletes who exercise so strenuously that they stop menstruating may be at risk for bone loss.

> In one of the first studies to demonstrate this finding, 25 young female athletes who had stopped menstruating for no apparent reason had 28% less bone mass than a comparison group of 45 women. The athletes typically have low estrogen levels.

BEGINNING AN EXERCISE PROGRAM

If you have been sedentary for more than one year, you should start with a visit to your doctor for a physical examination. This is to ensure that you don't have any symptomless conditions that could limit the type and amount of exercise you do.

If you are over age 45 you should also have an exercise stress test, in which your heart rate, blood pressure and possibly your breathing are monitored as you exercise on a treadmill or stationary bicycle. The doctor can then determine your overall fitness level, maximum heart rate and endurance level, information that is essential for designing the right program for you. The test can also help determine whether you have any signs of heart disease, a factor that should be taken into account before beginning any exercise program.

If you are a beginner, we recommend that you spend the first month or two strengthening your muscles. By doing so, you will be less likely to become injured when you begin the aerobic part of the program.

Then start adding aerobics. This includes walking, treadmill, stationary (recumbant) bicycle or Stairmaster. (If you have osteopenia or osteoporosis, you should be cautious in doing step aerobics; and be sure to use caution, good shoes and good body mechanics if you choose to ride a bicycle.)

Cardiovascular fitness. The guidelines outlined below will let you achieve cardiovascular fitness in 3 to 6 months.

- With any type of exercise, you must start each session slowly, with at least 5 minutes of warm-up exercises.

- The objective is to exercise to the point that your heart is working in the range from 70% to 85% of its capacity (your target zone) for at least 20 minutes and preferably for 30–45 minutes. As you exercise, check your pulse rate periodically to make sure you stay in the target zone.

- Maintain your pulse rate in the target zone for 20 minutes at least 3 times/week; 5 times/week would be better. (If you are below your target zone, push a little harder. If you are above your target zone, slow down.)

- End with cool-down exercises until your breathing rate and pulse have returned to normal.

To take your pulse: Stop exercising briefly, place two fingers along your carotid artery (at the side of your neck). Count the beats for 6 seconds (you'll need a clock with a second hand). Now multiply that number by 10 to get beats per minute (pulse rate).

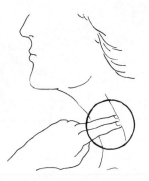

To find your maximum heart rate. This is a rough formula: subtract your age from the number 220.

To find your target zone. Multiply your maximum heart rate by .70 (for lower end of zone) and by .85 (for upper end of zone).

> *Example*: a woman has a maximum heart rate of 185 beats per minute (220-35=185). Her target zone is 129 beats per minute (70% of 185) to 157 beats per minute (85% of 185).

If you are over 45, this equation is less likely to be accurate— it may underestimate your target range. In that case you may not exercise to your full capacity or reap the full cardiovascular benefits. An exercise stress test can determine your maximum heart rate and target range.

An alternate way to find your target zone is use the chart below. Find your pulse on the left hand column, then find your age along the bottom. The area where they connect is your target zone. You can see from the chart how the target zone decreases with age.

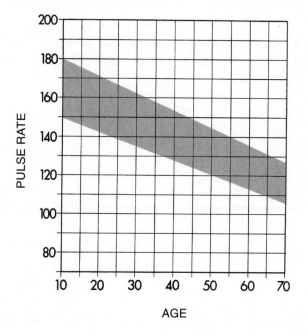

Recommendations   Even though any physical activity is good, a program of sustained moderate exercise for 3 to 5 times a week is ideal, both for your heart and your bones.

If you have been sedentary for more than a year or for some other reason simply can't manage 20 minutes or more of continuous physical activity, *any* increase in physical activity is better than none.

Several studies have shown that postmenopausal women who gain bone mass by exercising regularly lose it again after they stop. To maintain fitness—and bone health—you must continue exercising regularly for the rest of your life.

8 Drugs That Help Prevent Bone Loss & Increase Bone Mass

Prevention of bone loss is the ideal goal. Once bone is gone, treatment may strengthen the bone that remains but it cannot completely replace the bone architecture that has been lost.

Most of the available drugs help prevent bone loss and increase bone mass by *slowing down or stopping further bone loss;* they are called *antiresorptive.* Estrogen, calcitonin and bisphosphonates are antiresorptive agents.

- Antiresorptive drugs inhibit osteoclast activity, slowing down the bone removal process. The osteoblasts are not affected so new bone formation continues, thus leading to a net increase in bone mass.

Other drugs stimulate new bone formation. Sodium fluoride is the only available bone formation stimulant, although some studies suggest that androgens (when added to estrogen) may act as a bone stimulant, too.

123

- Bone remodeling stimulants create an increase in the amount of new bone formed that is greater than what is lost, resulting in a substantial increase in bone mass.

SHOULD YOU HAVE DRUG THERAPY?

Drug therapy could prevent osteoporosis in just about every woman after menopause. But because some risk does exist, it would not be medically or ethically desirable for doctors to treat everyone when only half of them will ultimately develop osteoporosis. Whether or not you should have treatment, therefore, is based on your personal risk for osteoporosis or, preferably, a bone density test and other tests.

Bone density tests that show that you have low bone mass or are losing bone rapidly—or lab tests that show an excess excretion of urinary collagen and calcium (reflecting an accelerated rate of bone loss)—are *absolute indications for therapy*.

If you do not have access to these tests (availability of bone densitometry is increasing rapidly but still relatively few women have access to it), you may need to decide on preventive therapy based on your risk factors for osteoporosis.

Generally speaking, the more risk factors you have (*see Chapter 4*), the more you stand to gain from therapy.

The choices. For over 50 years, estrogen has been *the* effective therapy for preventing bone loss in postmenopausal women. Now, women who are unable or unwilling to take estrogen have other options for preventing or treating osteoporosis. Research involving alternative approaches is ongoing, with results appearing regularly in medical journals and repeated in the lay media. The options are growing.

ESTROGEN

Ever since 1940, when Fuller Albright, MD, proposed a relationship between estrogen deficiency at menopause and bone loss, estrogen replacement therapy (ERT) has been used to stop the progression of bone loss in postmenopausal women.

ERT can slow and/or stop bone loss and bring about significant increases in bone density in menopausal and postmenopausal women, thus preventing fractures. Research shows that estrogen-treated women have 40 to 50% fewer wrist and hip fractures and 90% fewer vertebral fractures than untreated women. Simply put, estrogen builds bone mass. But it does not repair bone or reconstitute bone that has been lost.

ERT can prevent further bone loss even when started after age 70. It is FDA-approved for both prevention and treatment of osteoporosis.

Side effects in the doses currently prescribed are very infrequent and are usually due to known biologic effects of the hormone, (such as menstruation), or extreme sensitivity (such as breast tenderness and fluid retention on low-dose estrogen). A woman might have intolerance to the lactose-filler in certain oral estrogens, resulting in symptoms of lactose intolerance (such as bloating). Very rarely, there is a total intolerance to the hormone, which could result in headaches, visual disturbances and a worsening of certain other medical conditions, such as porphyria. Mental depression is a side effect occasionally reported from taking certain synthetic progestins.

How does estrogen affect bone mass? By interacting with other hormones, estrogen influences regulation of bone metabolism and hence bone mass in the following ways:

- Blocks the bone-dissolving action of *parathyroid hormone*;

- Stimulates activation of *vitamin D* (which increases both calcium absorption through the intestines and reabsorption of calcium through the kidneys);

- Appears to stimulate the thyroid gland to produce *calcitonin* (which protects bones from dissolving effects of parathyroid hormone and inhibits bone breakdown);

- Stimulates the liver to produce proteins that bind with the *adrenal hormones* in the blood and prevent their bone-dissolving effects.

Estrogen also reduces the frequency of the bone remodeling cycle, resulting in a 40% reduced risk of developing perforations in the delicate plates of trabecular bone (which compromise structural integrity and strength).

In addition, estrogen increases collagen in some parts of the body (notably the skin) and it is suspected of doing the same in bone. In bone, collagen forms the matrix that calcium crystals adhere to.

In short, estrogen increases calcium absorption and results in improved calcium balance.

How do we know?   The first controlled study was reported in 1976. This was a five-year study of surgically menopausal women, all within three years of their menopause. Half were given estrogen therapy and the rest placebos (inactive

Estrogen increases calcium absorption.

pills). At the end of five years, the placebo group had the 1–2% annual loss of bone mass typical of postmenopausal women, while the estrogen group actually gained a small amount of bone.

As a follow-up, the investigators then set out to determine how long their patients needed to remain on estrogen therapy to prevent bone loss. They found that women given estrogen for four years and no estrogen for the next four lost as much bone as those who

Women who began hormone therapy within 3 years after menopause had an increase in bone mass.

had received no estrogen at all! The women on estrogen for the full eight years showed little or no bone loss at all.

This study continued for another 15 years with the same result: a progressive increase in bone mass in the women who took estrogen (and significantly fewer vertebral fractures), and a continued decrease among those who did not.

A great many studies—too many to list—have confirmed these results and shown that estrogen therapy is equally effective in preventing bone loss following a natural menopause.

Dosage and administration   There is no evidence that one type of estrogen is more effective than another. The form used isn't important either, so long as it raises the level of estrogen circulating in the bloodstream the right amount (to at least 40–80 pg/dl [picograms of estrogen per deciliter of blood]).

Pills: the daily dosage required to prevent bone loss is quite low: as low as 0.3 mg of esterified estrogen (Estratab), 0.5 mg of micronized estradiol (Estrace) or 0.625 mg of conjugated equine estrogen (Premarin). The latter is about one-sixth the amount of estrogen contained in low-dose oral contraceptives.

For women with an intact uterus, the addition of a progestogen (to protect the endometrium) may also enhance the efficacy of ERT in increasing bone density.

In general, lower doses of estrogen and progestogen maintain bone density. Higher doses are usually needed to significantly increase bone density.

Patch: transdermal patches include Vivelle (applied twice a week) and Climara (applied once a week). Both preparations come in varying dosages. Studies have demonstrated that the patch (and pellet, below) preserves bone mass to the same extent as oral ERT and may even be able to raise bone mass in some women.

Pellets: surgically menopausal women respond well to treatment with estrogen pellets that are inserted into the fatty tissue underlying the skin of the lower abdomen or upper buttocks. A local anesthetic is used. The average dose is 25 mg every 6 months.

Cream: estrogen vaginal creams are not effective for this use.

BISPHOSPHONATES

Bisphosphonates are potent inhibitors of bone breakdown. These drugs are not new; they have been used to treat various bone diseases over the past 20 years. Earlier concerns that they also slowed bone mineralization have not been justified.

Alendronate (Fosamax) is the only bisphosphonate so far that is FDA-approved for osteoporosis prevention and treatment. It acts by coating the active borders of the osteoclasts, thus slowing down the bone removal process.

In the first two years of a large, six-year Early Postmenopausal Interventional Cohort (EPIC) study, women treated with Fosamax 5 mg increased bone mass at the spine by 3.46% and total hip by 1.85% compared to baseline. The women who did not receive Fosamax lost 1.78% of bone mass at the spine and 1.42% at the hip. The increases in bone density were comparable to women in the study who were treated with HRT. (Dropout rate due to side effects: 13.6% of women on HRT, 8.2% on alendronate, 5.4% in the placebo group.)

In a multi-center international study, researchers followed 2,027 women ages 55 to 80 who had porous bones and a history of spinal fractures. After three years, those taking Fosamax 10 mg had 51% fewer hip fractures, 47% fewer spinal fractures, and 48% fewer wrist fractures than the placebo group. Fosamax also reduced the incidence of total hospitalization by 20% (24.9% with Fosamax vs 30.4%). In the study, 10 mg of alendronate taken daily increased bone mass in the spine and hip by almost 9% and 6%, respectively.

Fosamax remains in bone, even after therapy is halted. An advantage of Fosamax over estrogen is that bone loss resumes as soon as estrogen is halted, but Fosamax remains in bone for years, and could be effective after treatment is stopped.

Side effects include stomach upsets in some users. For this reason, alendronate should be taken sitting up, with a glass of plain water the first thing in the morning, at least a half hour before the first meal of the day.

Etidronate (Didronel) is not presently FDA-approved for osteoporosis therapy though it is approved for treatment of another bone condition: Paget's disease. Still, doctors have been using it successfully and safely in clinical practice, to treat women with osteoporosis.

One study, involving 429 women with osteoporosis, found that the rate of vertebral fractures was reduced by one-half in women who took Didronel. Those who started with the lowest bone density of the spine had the lowest subsequent vertebral fracture rate: two-thirds less than the control group.

Didronel is available as pills taken in a dose of 400 mg for 2 weeks every three months.

Risedronate (Actonel) is not presently FDA-approved for prevention or treatment of osteoporosis.

In an 18-month study, 648 postmenopausal women with osteoporosis who took risedronate experienced an increase in bone density in their hips, spines and wrists. The drug did not cause any gastrointestinal side effects.

Other bisphosphonates currently under investigation include pamidronate and ibandronate. Because these drugs inhibit bone resorption at doses much lower than those that impair bone mineralization, it is possible that they can be taken continuously for long periods of time, with even less potential gastrointestinal side effects than alendronate.

CALCITONIN

Calcitonin is a hormone (extracted from salmon) that is effective in slowing bone loss and may increase bone density. It appears to help most when the problem is caused by increased calcium excretion, which indicates a high rate of bone turnover (activation of the bone remodeling cycle). There's also evidence that calcitonin stimulates new bone formation by osteoblasts.

Calcitonin is FDA-approved and may be prescribed either as a subcutaneous (under the skin) injection, given every other day or three times a week (depending on need), or as a nasal spray (Miacalcin). To self-administer the spray, the container is pumped to release a metered dose of calcitonin into a nostril. The usual daily dose is two "puffs," which is equivalent to 200 international units.

In some studies, calcitonin has been found to be at least as good as estrogen in slowing bone loss, but estrogen is still more effective in increasing bone mass.

In a two-year study, British researchers found that calcitonin injections were equally effective in slowing bone loss of the vertebrae as estrogen.

Claus Christiansen, MD, and his colleagues at the University of Copenhagen found that 208 women who used the spray and took extra calcium for two years had two-thirds fewer spinal and hip fractures than a control group.

Calcitonin also has pain-relieving properties. This is especially significant in the treatment of women who have recently fractured their vertebrae.

The main side effect is that, in about 10% of women, Miacalcin causes some nasal irritation. Other side effects may include back and/or joint pain, headache, loss of appetite, a metallic taste in the mouth, nausea and vomiting, and flushing of the face, ears and sometimes the upper body. Most of these symptoms are mild and don't last very long. Some elderly patients find the pump hard to press.

Calcitonin slows bone loss and relieves pain.

Some women may develop a resistance to the drug after prolonged use (two years or longer). This can be reduced with lower doses and by not using it continuously.

FLUORIDE

Controversy still exists as to whether the bone in women treated with regular (plain) sodium fluoride is normal in composition. Some scientists feel the newly formed bone is too brittle. There have been reports of increased hip fractures and of no decrease in spinal fractures, in spite of an increase in bone mass.

In a four-year study by Lawrence Riggs, MD, at the Mayo Clinic in Rochester, Minnesota, the rate of spinal fractures in a group of women taking regular sodium fluoride stayed the same, despite a 35% increase in spinal bone density.

Fluoride is incorporated into bone during the mineralization stage, but because it alters the size and structure of the bone crystals, it is thought to decrease the mechanical strength of the bone (it may cause collagen fibers to be laid down in a disorganized fashion). It can also impair bone mineralization in women whose calcium and vitamin D intake is low.

On the other hand, studies (and clinical practice) have shown that when low-dose plain fluoride is used together with calcium, vitamin D and/or estrogen, it can substantially increase bone density *and* prevent fractures. This was confirmed most recently by Charles Pak, MD, using a specially formulated slow-release form of sodium fluoride. This formulation differs in composition from regular sodium fluoride.

In Dr. Pak's studies, slow-release sodium fluoride, supplemented with calcium, was shown to build new bone and prevent spinal fractures in postmenopausal women with osteoporosis. But so far this therapy has not been approved by the FDA to treat osteoporosis.

Since fluoride is the only drug that promotes significant new bone formation, some researchers (including ourselves) believe that slow-release sodium fluoride-with-estrogen may be the key to successful bone-building therapy. Estrogen increases bone matrix prior to mineralization, and calcium and sodium fluoride can properly mineralize the bone.

Slow-release sodium fluoride with estrogen may be the key to successful bone building therapy.

Side effects from high doses of plain fluoride include gastrointestinal problems such as stomach pain, nausea, vomiting, diarrhea and gastrointestinal bleeding, occasional tenderness around the ankle, knee or hip, foot pain and joint stiffness. Newer, sustained-release forms of sodium fluoride are producing fewer side effects.

Although regular sodium fluoride is available over-the-counter, you should not use it except under a doctor's supervision.

ANDROGENS AND ANABOLIC STEROIDS

As mentioned earlier, androgens have been shown to slow down a loss in bone mass in a manner similar to estrogen. The biggest drawback has been the side effects, which include unwanted growth of facial and body hair, acne and deepening of the voice. These can be almost totally eliminated by adding estrogen to the therapy.

We found that women who took an androgen-estrogen combination (Estratest) increased their bone mass, while those on estrogen alone simply maintained bone mass.

In a more recent study, Estratest increased bone density of the spine more than 1.25 mg of Premarin.

A new synthetic steroid, known in the U.S. as OD-14 (Tibilone), also shows promise of becoming yet another option. The drug has properties of androgens, progesterone and estrogen. Studies in Europe have shown that the drug actually slows bone loss, increases bone mass, and reduces the risk of fractures in osteoporosis patients.

Anabolic steroids have been found to increase bone mass, as well. One such steroid, Durabolin, is currently being used in Europe for the management of severe osteopenia and osteoporosis.

VITAMIN D

Calcitriol is a very potent form of an activated vitamin D, given in pill form. It has been shown to increase bone mass in women with osteoporosis, and is believed to work by slowing down bone resorption (breakdown) and helping the body retain calcium. It is the most frequently used therapy for osteoporosis in Japan. But so far it has not been approved for use in the U.S.

Because it can raise blood calcium levels, it can cause kidney stones. Most otherwise healthy women with osteoporosis will probably do as well with regular vitamin D supplements prescribed in doses of 600 to 800 mg per day.

THIAZIDE DIURETICS

These drugs, which are widely used to treat high blood pressure, decrease the amount of calcium excreted in the urine. Not surprisingly, some researchers have found that thiazides appear to increase or at least preserve bone density in older women.

Results from the Framingham Heart Study, the well-known survey of more than 5,000 people (average age 68), begun in the 1940s and still ongoing, found that women who took thiazide diuretics had one-third fewer hip fractures.

Two other studies (one at the University of Florida, one reported by Honolulu researchers), confirmed the conclusions of the Framingham studies.

SERMs

There are a number of synthetic drugs being developed that are individually designed to give the benefits of estrogen without the risks. They are called Selective Estrogen Receptor Modulators (SERMs), and are referred to as "designer estrogens" or "anti-estrogens." The results look promising. However, it will be years before all the true risks and benefits are known.

Tamoxifen (Nolvadex) is commonly used in the treatment of estrogen-dependent breast cancer. It works by blocking the natural action of estrogen on breast tissue. It also inhibits bone breakdown and preserves bone mass. In women receiving tamoxifen for the treatment of breast cancer, bone of the lumbar spine is preserved and even increases.

Like any drug, there are side effects. Women may experience hot flashes, headaches, vaginal discharge and irregular menstruation. Depression is another possible side effect, as well as a slightly increased risk for an aggresive form of endometrial cancer. Annual monitoring of the endometrium is advised *(see page 149)*.

Raloxifene (Evista) is a close cousin of tamoxifen and has the same bone-mineral enhancing effect. It appears to exhibit some of the positive effects of estrogen, including an antiresorptive effect in bone, and a cholesterol lowering effect. Unlike estrogen, raloxifene does not stimulate the uterine lining (endometrium), and behaves as an anti-estrogen in breast tissue.

It's too soon to know if raloxifene protects the coronary arteries in the heart. In a recent study in monkeys, it failed to prevent plaque formation in the coronary arteries, whereas estrogen (Premarin) did.

Side effects seen in some women include blood clots in the legs and hot flashes. Almost 30% of women in the clinical trial complained of hot flashes.

In clinical trials on 1,200 postmenopausal women ages 45 to 65, three-fourths took raloxifene (various doses), the rest had a placebo. Researchers found that the women on raloxifene (60 mg/day) increased bone density by a modest 1.5% after two years of treatment, while those on the placebo lost bone (1%). Subjects on estrogen (Premarin) increased their bone density by 2.5% to 3%.

In other, comparable, studies, women on HRT (Premarin and Provera) increased bone density by 5.2%, and women on alendronate for two years imcreased bone density by an average of 5.8%.

A new study of raloxifene—7,700 women, ages 60 to 75, in 20 countries—will examine spine fracture, breast cancer, strokes, heart attacks, mental acuity, and side effects.

The results of this study will help to place its role into a more realistic perspective. (It should be noted that the protective effect of Tamoxifen on breast cancer is significantly reduced after five years of use.)

Other SERMs   Additional SERMs in current research include droloxifene (Pfizer) and levomeloxifene (Novo Nordisk). Clinical date is not yet available on these preparations. Researchers will continue to study this promising new treatment for osteoporosis, to assess the medication's long-term effects.

PARATHYROID HORMONE

Scientists are investigating whether parathyroid hormone (PTH), given intermittently in low doses, stimulates the building of bone. (In high doses it can stimulate bone breakdown.)

> In one study, 50 women on estrogen therapy were given daily injections of PTH. The women showed dramatic increases of bone mass in the spine, averaging 13%, and smaller increases at the hip and the rest of the skeleton.

GROWTH FACTORS

Scientists are testing the effects of growth factors as possible stimulants to bone formation. It will probably be many years before this type of therapy becomes practical for patient use.

DRUG COMBINATIONS

Since there are a number of drugs that preserve bone via slightly differing mechanisms, it seems likely that a combination would do even more than single drug therapy. It is too early to know which drug combinations are best. The only published data show that an estrogen/etidronate combination has an additive effect on bone mass.

PHYTOESTROGENS

Phytoestrogens, or "plant estrogens" (for example, genistene) derived from soybeans, and so-called bioflavanoids (ipriflavone) comprise a new class of drugs derived from plants that holds promise as an option for preventing and treating osteoporosis.

These substances suppress bone breakdown without affecting the uterine lining or increasing the risk of endometrial cancer. Nor do they carry any risk of breast cancer. In preliminary studies, women had a reduction in cholesterol and small increases in bone mineral density in the spine. More research on larger groups of women needs to be done before recommendations can be made.

PREPARATIONS FOR PREVENTION AND/OR TREATMENT
OF OSTEOPOROSIS

ESTROGEN (ORAL)

BRAND NAME	NAME OF DRUG/HORMONE	MANUFACTURER
Congest d	conjugated estrogen	Trianon
C.S.D. d	conjugated estrogen	Pharmascience
Estinyl d	conjugated estrogen	Schering
Estrace	micronized estradiol	Bristol-Myers Squibb
Estratab	esterified estrogen	Solvay
Menest e	esterified estrogen	Beecham
Neo-Estrone d	conjugated estrogen	Neolab
Ogen	estropipate	Upjohn
Ortho-Est d	estropipate	Ortho
Premarin	conjugated equine estrogen	Wyeth-Ayerst

ESTROGEN (PATCH)

BRAND NAME	NAME OF DRUG/HORMONE	MANUFACTURER
Alora	estradiol	Proctor & Gamble
Climara	estradiol	Berlex
Estraderm	estradiol	Ciba
Vivelle	estradiol	Ciba

ESTROGEN (INJECTION)

BRAND NAME	NAME OF DRUG/HORMONE	MANUFACTURER
Delestrogen	estradiol	Bristol-Myers Squibb

ESTROGEN-PROGESTOGEN COMBINATION (ORAL)

BRAND NAME	NAME OF DRUG/HORMONE	MANUFACTURER
PremPro	conjugated estrogens/	
PremPhase	medroxyprogesterone acetate	Wyeth-Ayerst

PROGESTRONE

BRAND NAME	NAME OF DRUG/HORMONE	MANUFACTURER
Prometrium	micronized progesterone	Solvay

a - in clinical research
b - not FDA approved
c - not named yet
d - available in Canada only
e - available in U.S. only

PROGESTOGEN

BRAND NAME	NAME OF DRUG/HORMONE	MANUFACTURER
Amen [e]	medroxyprogesterone acetate	Carnrick
.Aygestin [e]	norethindrone acetate	Wyeth-Ayerst
Colprone [d]	medrogestone	Wyeth-Ayerst
Cycrin [e]	medroxyprogesterone acetate	ESI-Pharma
Megace	megestrol acetate	Bristol-Myers Squibb
Micronor	norethindrone	Ortho
Norlutate	norethindrone acetate	Parke-Davis
Nor-QD [e]	norethindrone	Syntex
Ovrette [e]	norgestrel	Wyeth-Ayerst
PMS-Progesterone [d]	progesterone	Pharmascience
Provera	medroxyprogesterone acetate	Upjohn

BISPHOSPHONATES

BRAND NAME	NAME OF DRUG/HORMONE	MANUFACTURER
Fosamax	alendronate	Merck & Co.
Didronel	etidronate	Procter & Gamble
Actonel	residronate	Proctor & Gamble
b c	ibandronate	Boehrenger-Mannheim

ESTROGEN AGONIST/ANTAGONISTS (SERMs)

BRAND NAME	NAME OF DRUG/HORMONE	MANUFACTURER
Nolvadex	tamoxifen	Zeneca
Evista	raloxifene	Eli Lilly
a c	droloxifene	Pfizer
a c	levomeloxifene	Novo Nordisk

CALCITONIN

BRAND NAME	NAME OF DRUG/HORMONE	MANUFACTURER
Miacalcin	calcitonin (nasal spray)	Sandoz

FLUORIDE

BRAND NAME	NAME OF DRUG/HORMONE	MANUFACTURER
b c	slow-release sodium fluoride	Mission Pharm.

9 Pros and Cons of Estrogen Therapy

Despite the fact that estrogen receptors (found in all tissues in the body) are essential for reproductive and general health, hormone therapy for postmenopausal women has long been controversial. Research continues to look for definitive answers.

So far, in spite of the potential risks associated with estrogen (as indeed there is with any therapy), most experts agree that for most women the benefits far outweigh the risks. Estrogen is routinely prescribed for women who have a high risk of osteoporosis, and physicians with experience in prescribing hormone replacement therapy believe it should be offered to most women.

BENEFITS OF ESTROGEN

Estrogen's bone-building effects have been well-documented. Studies have shown that it cuts the risk of hip fractures up to 50% if treatment begins at menopause and may help even when treatment begins at 70 or older.

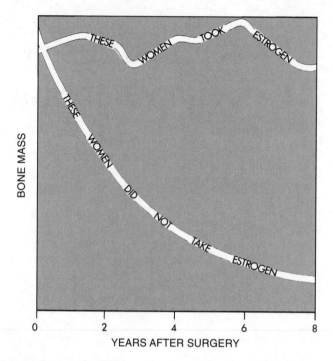

PREVENTION OF BONE LOSS WITH ESTROGEN THERAPY. Women who took estrogen after a surgical menopause did not lose bone. Those who took a placebo lost large amounts of bone.

After a surgical menopause, women who took estrogen did not lose bone; those in the placebo group lost large amounts of bone.

Estrogen has other benefits as well:

Life span Research has shown that postmenopausal women on ERT live longer.

In a study by Bruce Ettinger, MD, of Kaiser Permanente in Oakland, California, women who took estrogen for 5 or more years had a 46% reduced risk of dying from all causes. Those who used the hormone for 15 or more years reduced their risk of death by about half over nonusers.

Epidemiologist Francine Grodstein and her colleagues at Brigham and Women's Hospital in Boston collected data on 38,000 women participating in Harvard Medical

School's Nurses Health Study. They found that women who took ERT were 37% less likely to have died than those not on the hormone.

Heart disease   A major benefit of ERT is estrogen's protective role against heart disease. Almost every research study has concluded that ERT reduces the risk of coronary artery disease by about 40% to 50% This is true even if you have other risk factors for heart disease, such as high blood pressure, elevated cholesterol levels or obesity.

Researchers see the greatest benefits in long-term use. Estrogen helps lower levels of "bad" LDL cholesterol and raise "good" HDL cholesterol—one reason premenopausal women have a much lower rate of heart disease than their male peers. In addition, ERT improves insulin metabolism (a factor in causing atherosclerosis) and prevents spasm of the coronary arteries.

Alzheimer's disease   Recent studies show that ERT can reduce a woman's risk of developing Alzheimer's by 30% to 40%. And evidence is growing that women who already have Alzheimer's will gain improved mental abilities, especially verbal memory.

In a five-year study of 1,124 women age 70 and over, Columbia University researchers found that the longer the women took estrogen, the lower their risk of developing Alzheimer's. And in cases where estrogen did not prevent Alzeimer's, it appeared to delay its onset by several years.

More recently, another study showed that the risk of Alzheimer's was reduced by more than 50% among hormone users.

ERT = estrogen replacement therapy (estrogen alone). Used most commonly in women who have had a hysterectomy. Taken daily.

HRT = hormone replacement therapy (estrogen + a progestogen). Prescribed for women with an intact uterus. The estrogen is taken daily. The progestogen can be taken cyclically, e.g., 12-14 days a month, or daily.

Memory   Estrogen is believed to improve memory in post-menopausal women. This finding adds to a growing body of evidence that estrogen can benefit the aging brain.

Colon cancer   Two recent studies published in the Journal of the National Cancer Institute found that among ERT users, the risk of colon cancer was cut almost in half .

Teeth and gums   Women who take estrogen supplements have healthier teeth and gums.

> A recent study of 300 women between ages 50 and 74 found that those taking estrogen had less bone loss around the teeth, less gum bleeding, and more of their own teeth than women not on estrogen.

Cataracts   At least three recent studies suggest that estrogen therapy may have a protective effect on the eye. Potential advantages include improved lens transmittance and a decrease in frequency of lens opacities, including cataracts. This benefit appears to accrue with long-term ERT. The data is still preliminary but it does appear that women on ERT for osteoporosis prevention will note an additional benefit for their eyes.

Wrinkling   Belgian researchers found that postmenopausal women who took ERT had skin that was almost as taut as that of premenopausal women. But ERT will not negate wrinkling due to sun damage.

WHAT ARE THE RISKS?

Does estrogen increase a woman's risk of developing cancer of the breast and uterus? Here's a closer look at these and other potential risks associated with estrogen.

Cancer of the uterus   Over a long period of time, estrogen can overstimulate the endometrium (lining of the uterus). If untreated, this can lead to endometrial cancer. But how great is the risk?

In women who don't take estrogen, the expected incidence of endometrial cancer in one year is 1 in 1,000. When estrogen is used alone (ERT) it can increase the risk from 2 times to 13 times. While a thirteenfold increase sounds alarming, it should be placed in perspective. Each year there are 5,700 deaths from endometrial cancer (not all of these are a result of estrogen therapy); now compare this with approximately *50,000 deaths from hip fractures.*

While the potential risk of endometrial cancer is not to be taken lightly, if is detected and treated in its earliest (precancerous) stages it is virtually 100% curable. Moreover, the type that develops in estrogen users has a higher cure rate than other types. You should be monitored by your physician and undergo yearly screening tests *(see pages 146–147).*

Removing the risk. Any risk at all is not necessary. If you take estrogen plus a *progestogen* (synthetic form of progesterone) for at least 10 days every month, the endometrium is protected—*the risk of developing endometrial cancer is even lower than it is in women who do not take any hormones at all!* Current evidence suggests that estrogen's protective effect against heart disease remains.

In the 1995 PEPI (Postmenopausal Estrogen/Progestin Interventions) study conducted by the National Institutes of Health, 875 healthy women taking daily HRT for three years had increases in bone density in both spine and hip. The women were divided into five groups: (1) estrogen alone, (2) estrogen + progestogen, (3) estrogen + cyclical progestogen, (4) estrogen + cyclical natural progesterone, (5) placebo.

The placebo group lost about 2% bone density in the spine and hip. Those on HRT gained 3.5 to 5% bone density in the spine and nearly 2% in the hip.

Adding a progestogen did not affect estrogen's beneficial effect on cardiovascular risk factors. Both estrogen and combination therapy lowered LDL cholesterol by about 20%. Protective HDL cholesterol rose in users of hormone therapy and dropped somewhat in non-hormone users.

To overcome the menstruation "side effect." Your physician will probably prescribe a progestogen for you to take for at least 10 to 14 days every month to protect against endometrial cancer. The downside is that you may have menstrual-like bleeding each time you stop the progestogen. This is an inconvenience most women accept when they understand why it is so important. *If you bleed at any other time or notice a change in the amount of flow, you should notify your physician at once.*

Some physicians prescribe low doses of both estrogen and progestogen to be taken daily without interruption. A new trend involves taking progestogen for 2 weeks every 3 months. The available data suggest that these methods protect the endometrium as well as the other methods.

Breast cancer   Estrogen receptors in breast tissue create the means for estrogen to be linked to breast cancer. Even your own natural estrogen has an effect.

Various factors increase or decrease your risk:

- A long menstrual life, characterized by early onset of menstruation (before age 12) and/or a late menopause (after age 55) increases your risk.

- Your age when you had your first pregnancy: before age 20 reduces your risk; after age 30 increases it.

- Multiple pregnancies seem somewhat protective.

- Surgical removal of the ovaries before age 35 gives protection. (Whether or not ERT after a surgical menopause negates this protective effect is not known.)

It is important to understand that estrogen doesn't *cause* breast cancer. But it may encourage the growth of some kinds of already-existing cancer cells. Estrogen will also double your risk if you have a family history of the disease. (However, you may be surprised to know that in the 1970s, estrogen was used to treat breast cancer and, for certain cancers, actually enhanced the cure rate!)

The estrogen-breast cancer scare was first fueled by a highly publicized 1989 Swedish study. Those on a combination of estrogen and progestogen had about 10% more breast cancer than expected. Of the women on estrogen for nine years or more, the incidence increased to 70% above expected levels.

Two recent U.S. studies came to opposite conclusions. *One declared that ERT contributed to the risk of breast cancer; the other said it did not!* Both studies were widely covered by the media, resulting in confusion and then distrust regarding the safety of estrogen.

Recently, a thorough analysis of well-designed studies on this subject found that postmenopausal estrogen users face only a slight increased risk of the disease. After 15 years, the risk (not the number of cases) may increase by about 30%, which would mean only 3 more cases per 10,000 women.

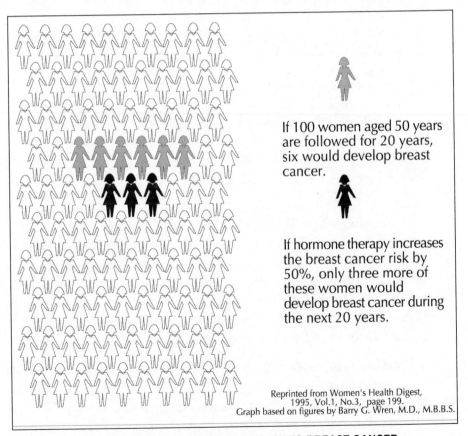

If 100 women aged 50 years are followed for 20 years, six would develop breast cancer.

If hormone therapy increases the breast cancer risk by 50%, only three more of these women would develop breast cancer during the next 20 years.

Reprinted from Women's Health Digest, 1995, Vol.1, No.3, page 199.
Graph based on figures by Barry G. Wren, M.D., M.B.B.S.

RELATIONSHIP OF HORMONE THERAPY TO BREAST CANCER

According to Barry G. Wren, MD, professor of gynecology at the University of Sydney (Australia), if you followed one hundred 50-year-old women for 20 years, 6 would get breast cancer. If ERT increased this risk by 50% (which it does not), only 3 more would develop breast cancer.

Overall, for women with no family history of breast cancer, most of the current evidence suggests that postmenopausal estrogen therapy either has no effect on the risk of breast cancer or that it causes only a slightly elevated risk with very long-term use (more than 15 years) at relatively high doses. Taken for up to five years, it doesn't seem to raise the risk at all.

At this point, we believe that the proven benefits of protection from osteoporosis and heart disease clearly outweigh the possible slightly increased risk of breast cancer for the majority of women.

> *What is your risk?* The American Cancer Society estimates that 1 out of every 8 American women will develop breast cancer during her lifetime. It's a frightening thought. But they are describing a *lifetime risk*. At ages 40–59 it's only 1 in 26, rising at ages 60–79 to 1 in 15. It is still unresolved whether ERT after menopause (when estrogen levels are low and your risk of cancer naturally rises with age) increases the risk of breast cancer.

Weight gain   Donna Kritz-Silverstein, PhD and Elizabeth Barrett-Connor, MD of the University of California, San Diego, examined data from 671 women between the ages of 65 and 94 and found that, for those who had taken HRT for 15 years or more, there was no link between changes in body weight and the use of hormones. In fact, HRT actually redistributes the concentration of abdominal fat to the healthier female site of the thighs.

Other concerns   Early studies of young women who used oral contraceptives suggested that estrogen increased the risk of high blood pressure, thrombosis (blood clots) and cardiovascular disease. That raised concerns that postmenopausal estrogen therapy might do the same for older women, whose risk of these health problems naturally rises with age.

We now know, that is not the case. Those findings were based on high doses of hormones; birth control pills are now low-dose (they actually protect against heart disease), and the *estrogen in ERT is only one-sixth of that amount.* There is research evidence that estrogen therapy may actually lower blood pressure, and there is no cause-and-effect relationship between estrogen and the development of blood clots.

WHO SHOULD NOT TAKE ESTROGEN

Your risk factors or medical history may preclude the use of ERT under any circumstances. Or you may be able to use ERT cautiously under strict medical observation. These guidelines may help:

Do not take estrogen if you . . .

- Have had an estrogen-dependent breast cancer.
- Have had a recent blood-clotting disorder.

Do not take <u>oral</u> estrogen if you . . .

- Are a heavy smoker (other forms may be more effective).
- Have a disease involving the liver or gallbladder or have high blood levels of triglycerides (sugar fat). (Forms of estrogen that bypass the liver, such as the estrogen patch, are safe to use).

In the following situations you probably should not be on estrogen, but if you completely understand the risks and are closely monitored by a physician, you may be able to take estrogen if you . . .

- Have a family history of breast cancer.
- Have ever had side effects from estrogen therapy or oral contraceptives.

Ask your doctor whether you can consider estrogen . . .

- If you have had endometrial cancer. HRT may be safe, depending on the stage and severity of the cancer. (Women with a history of cervical and certain types of ovarian cancer may also be able to take estrogen.)

- If you have had a melanoma, the most serious form of skin cancer. It is still not clear whether or not estrogen encourages its growth.

- If you have high blood presssure, coronary heart disease or diabetes. You will need to be closely monitored by your physician. Given the beneficial effect estrogen has on these conditions, many physicians (the authors included) regard them to be actual indications for ERT.

IF YOU DECIDE TO TAKE ESTROGEN

To be most effective, therapy should begin within five years of menopause, to prevent the large bone losses that occur during this period. Most women have a 4–7% *increase* in bone density within two years after starting estrogen therapy, which then levels off after two to three years.

Therapy initiated five to six years after menopause will still slow loss of bone, but it is less likely to restore density to premenopausal levels because too much bone has

The earlier you begin ERT, the better off you'll be.

already been lost. In other words, the earlier you begin therapy, the better off you'll be; but it is never too late to begin.

Bone loss may resume after you stop taking estrogen. So if you have significant osteopenia or osteoporosis, we recommend that you continue taking hormones for the rest of your life, provided you have no contraindications to the drug or experience any serious side effects.

While you are taking estrogen, remember to follow the other guidelines for protecting your bones: eat properly and exercise regularly. Take at least 1,000 mg of calcium and 400–600 IU of vitamin D daily, and watch out for the "bone robbers" (*chapter 6*).

Precautions you should take　　If you decide to take estrogen, you will be on therapy for a long time, and there are certain precautions you must take.

- Before you begin therapy, have a complete physical, including Pap smear, pelvic and breast exams, and mammogram. You should repeat these exams once a year while you are on estrogen therapy.

- Check your breasts at home *once a week.* As you become familiar with your breasts you will be better able to detect any *unfamiliar* lumps.

- Have your blood pressure checked every 6 months and alert your doctor (if someone else does does the checking) if it gets higher. Your physician may also recommend glucose and cholesterol tests.

- If your uterus is intact, you should be taking a progestogen to protect against endometrial cancer. You should also have *endometrial sampling (see below).*

- Ideally, you should have an annual bone density test to determine how well the therapy is working. Lab tests can show if the estrogen is being absorbed and if your bone density is responding to treatment.

Endometrial sampling. This test may be done before starting therapy, to determine if there are any precancerous cells in the uterus that could be stimulated by estrogen. Or you could wait three months, to see how the uterine lining responds to the hormones.

The test usually takes place in the doctor's office. A speculum is placed in the vagina to expose the cervix, and a suctioning instrument is inserted through the cervix into the uterus. (Your doctor may inject a local anesthetic into the cervix to help dilate it and ease cramping.) Samples of the uterine lining are removed for examination under a microscope.

Most women experience temporary pain that they describe as "like menstrual cramps." Much of this cramping can be prevented by taking a prostaglandin-inhibiting drug (used for relief of menstrual cramps) an hour before and again several hours afterward.

If your cervix cannot be dilated, or if you are extremely sensitive to pain, there is an alternative—ultrasound can be used to measure the thickness of your uterine lining. Ultrasound can be done either abdominally (by moving a probe slowly over your abdomen) or vaginally (by inserting the probe gently into the vagina).

What if estrogen doesn't work? Continued bone loss may be an indication that, for some reason, your body is not absorbing the estrogen. This happens to 10% to 20% of women taking oral estrogen, depending on the type and dose prescribed. It is one reason why it is so important to be monitored by your physician.

Case report: Barbara, age 54

Barbara was doing all the right things to protect her bones. She was on oral postmenopausal estrogen therapy. Every day she took 1,450 milligrams of calcium and 500 IU of vitamin D, and she followed an excellent exercise program consisting of brisk 45-minute walks 3 times a week and tennis 3 times a week.

But her second bone density test revealed that she was continuing to lose bone in the hip, putting her at risk for a hip fracture.

A check of Barbara's blood estrogen level showed that the estrogen she was taking was, in fact, being absorbed by her body. However, the level of follicle stimulating hormone in the bloodstream (released from the pituitary gland to stimulate the ovaries) was four times as high as it should have been, indicating that the estrogen she was taking was not biologically active (probably a result of its being bound by proteins as it passed through the liver).

Barbara was advised to switch to a non-oral type of estrogen, such as the estrogen skin patch.

If you decide not to take estrogen To prevent osteoporosis, experts agree that a woman's best weapon is three-pronged: increased calcium, weight-resistance exercises, and estrogen taken for at least five years. For the vast majority of women, the overall benefits of ERT (including enhanced quality of life, protection against heart disease and Alzheimer's disease) outweigh the relatively small risk of an ERT-related breast cancer.

If you do not choose to take estrogen, for any reason, you may want to discuss with your doctor the possibility of trying one of the other drug therapies now being used to prevent osteoporosis.

10 If You Already Have Osteoporosis

The worst has happened. A bone fractured. Or, you have not seen any visible sign of osteoporosis (nothing has fractured), but your bone density test reveals that your bone mass is so low it is defined as osteoporosis.

Now what?

IF YOUR TEST SAYS "OSTEOPOROSIS"

After the shocking truth has sunk in, you probably have many questions.

Was the test accurate?

Could the doctor be wrong?

Should I have a second opinion?

What can I take to cure it?

How could this have happened to me?

Though you may have heard the term osteoporosis from time to time, this may be the first time you have given serious thought to the problem. But if you have already lost more than 30% of peak bone mass, or if you have low bone mass along with one or more fractures, you have osteoporosis.

Fortunately, there are ways to prevent further bone loss.

Women who have significant osteopenia will benefit from treatment just as those with actual osteoporosis. "Treatment" is a bit of a misnomer, as osteopenia and osteoporosis are not diseases that can be treated, cured and forgotten.

Fortunately, you can prevent further bone loss.

"Management" is perhaps a better term, since therapy must be continued until such time as there is a natural slowing of bone loss. Recent research indicates that even women over age 70 continue to lose bone mass. Therefore, this frequently translates into lifelong therapy.

IF YOU'VE HAD A VERTEBRAL FRACTURE

Severe localized back pain of sudden onset should make you suspect that one of your spinal bones has fractured. You need to seek medical attention right away.

Your physician will probably recommend a narcotic, such as Demerol or Vicodan, to help relieve the acute pain. Once the pain has subsided somewhat, you may be able to use a milder product, such as Tylenol with codeine or Fiorinal. Antispasmodic drugs may be prescribed to help relieve muscle spasms, and if pain is severe ice packs over the fracture may help. A back brace is an option for helping to ease muscle pain during the first few weeks after the fracture. Certain medications (e.g., calcitonin) can immediately begin to strengthen the bone, speed its healing, and relieve the pain.

A few days of bed rest may be recommended. If it is, lie flat on your back or on your side; do not sit or get into a semi-reclining position. Standing is okay. Physical

Avoid sitting if you've had a spinal fracture.

therapist Sara Meeks suggests "active" bed rest—isometric strengthening exercises you can do while on your back *(exercises 1–4 beginning on page 162).*

If back pain persists for more than 12 weeks after the vertebra has healed, it is probably caused by muscle tension and muscle spasms related to the change in your posture.

Physical therapy to strengthen the back muscles that hold the spine erect is more effective and long-lasting than drugs or back braces. It's best to start therapy early. Proper exercises can help prevent the postural component of

Proper exercises can strengthen the muscles that hold the spine erect.

the humped back that develops in women with osteoporotic spinal fractures.

The 10 exercises that begin on page 162 are designed for this purpose. You may also want to ask your doctor for a referral to a physical therapist experienced in treating osteoporosis.

HOW TO KEEP THE PROBLEM FROM GETTING WORSE

Although osteoporosis may have already caused a certain amount of physical deformity and disability, there are measures you can take to prevent further bone loss and substantially reduce your chances of suffering more fractures. No treatment can "uncollapse" a collapsed vertebra, but treatment can slow down the loss of bone, perhaps even halt it totally, and in some cases actually increase your bone mass. In addition, there are things you can do to help prevent falling *(see pages 175-178)*.

Many of the same nutritional and exercise strategies used for prevention are essential ingredients of a management program. As with prevention, the therapy consists of three parts: good nutrition, selective medication, and appropriate exercise.

Nutrition   Eating right is more important than ever. If you've never given thought to a proper diet, now is the time to change your thinking.

You should be getting 1,400 to 2,000 milligrams of calcium and 800 units of vitamin D every day. Because it is important for you to absorb as much of the calcium as possible, spread it out during the day—don't take more than 500 mg of elemental calcium at one time, and take it with a little milk or orange juice. Be wary of

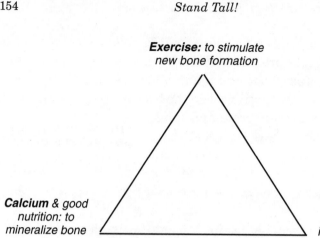

THREE ELEMENTS OF BONE HEALTH

the "bone robbers": large amounts of protein, red meat, coffee, salt, fiber, oxalates and phytates.

If you are a smoker, try to stop. This is no time for drinking too much either, as alcohol can prevent you from absorbing the calcium you desparately need and, by causing liver damage, may also impair your body's ability to produce activated vitamin D. Drinking can also cause you to lose your balance and fall, thereby increasing your risk of suffering a debilitating hip fracture.

Posture and body mechanics   If you have sustained one or more spinal fractures, or even if your test shows that you have low bone mass, it is especially important for you to stand (and sit) tall and practice good posture. Slumping your shoulders can exacerbate the muscle tension and pain triggered by the fracture. Poor posture can also affect your balance. General conditioning exercises and muscle-strengthening exercises for the upper body and back can help improve your posture.

Because a spinal fracture can result from even the minor exertions of everyday living—lifting a child or opening a window, for example—it is essential for you to practice good body mechanics. This means learning how to stand up, sit down, lift and reach, to accommodate your back and help maintain your balance.

Sitting or standing with good posture involves keeping your upper body aligned with your hips. One way to assure that your trunk is aligned with your hips, according to physical therapist Vibeke Vala, a consultant to the National Osteoporosis Foundation, is to take a deep breath, tighten your pelvic floor muscles (the muscles that control bladder and bowels) and pull in your stomach and lower abdomen. Try to do this every time you get out of bed or move from a sitting to a standing position.

You can learn how to stand, sit, lift and reach without doing harm.

Exercise   No matter how serious your condition, you will not get better unless you get moving. Exercise builds bone mass. But the amount of exercise needed to maximize bone growth is not known. Remember, your bone was lost over a long period of time. Work slowly but progressively at building it back up again. Exercise also strengthens muscles and improves coordination, which can help keep you from falling.

It is important to keep a balance between exercise that is beneficial and that which is overly strenuous. Overdoing could cause fracturing. Be wary of exercises or movements that compress the spine. *Research has shown that people with osteoporosis who perform flexion exercises are at a significant risk for fracture.*

Walking. Highly recommended for most people who have osteoporosis, walking is weightbearing and is not likely to harm the skeleton. It is important for you to walk with good alignment and body mechanics *(see page 116).*

Because walking is not strenuous, you should do it twice a day; once in the morning to limber up and again in the evening. If you are in fair to poor physical condition, begin with a 5-minute walk, preferably in an area with some slopes. Move along at a brisk pace. Add 1 minute each week, gradually building up to 20 minutes.

Jogging and running. Because they cause jarring to the skeleton, jogging and running may not be appropriate. Consult your physician first. Some women with previous healed osteoporosis may be able to participate in low-impact aerobics. If so, wear supportive shoes that help absorb the shock of impact. As with walking, use good alignment and body mechanics.

Working out. Good exercises in the gym include rowing (with

Good body mechanics for everyday activities

TO SIT DOWN. Bend knees to lower yourself onto the front edge of the chair. Use hands for support, to avoid "plopping" into the seat.

TO GET UP. Place one foot forward and scoot to the front of the seat. Use a rocking motion to stand up. Avoid "giving way" at the waist.

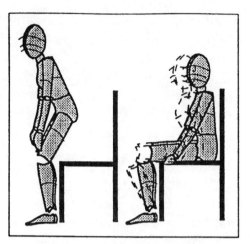

TO LIFT. Use your knees and legs instead of your back when lifting heavy objects.

Slide object up on one thigh and hold close at waist level with both hands before standing up.

Keep heavy objects close to your body (and your center of gravity) while lifting and carrying them.

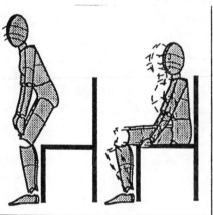

TO PICK UP BABY. Squat down and bring baby close before standing up. Use your knees and keep your back straight. If the child is old enough, sit down first and let him/her climb onto your lap.

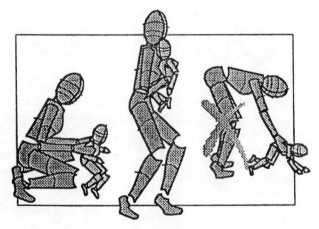

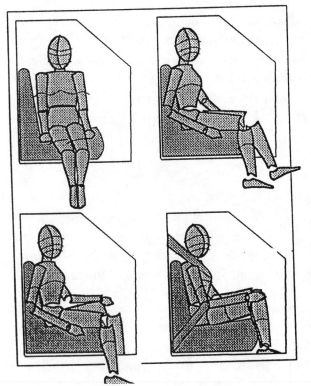

GETTING INTO THE CAR. Open the door and stand with your back to the opening. Sit down on the seat, then carefully move one leg, then the other, into the car.

GETTING OUT OF THE CAR. With the door open, turn your body and carefully place both legs outside of the car, then stand up with both feet firmly on the ground.

GETTING INTO BED. Lower yourself to lie down on one side by raising your legs and lowering your head at the same time. Use your arms to assist moving without twisting. Bend both knees to roll onto your back.

GETTING OUT OF BED. Roll onto your side. Push your upper body up with your arms while placing your feet over the side of the bed so that you are sitting on the edge of the bed. With your feet firmly on the floor, use your hands to push up to a standing position.

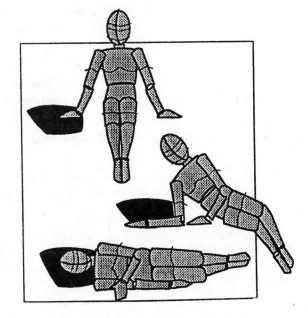

the back straight and emphasizing scapular [shoulder blade] movement), military presses, lateral arm raises (with back supported), and presses behind the neck. All of these exercises should be closely monitored by a trained exercise counselor or physical therapist.

Lat pulldowns, knee extensions or leg curls can be performed with caution—the back should be supported and you should be strong enough to maintain a neutral back position during the movement.

Avoid flexion (forward bending) movements or any resistive exercises that emphasize forward movements. Do not do abdom-**If you have osteoporosis and** inal crunches, leg lifts, knee-to-chest **do bending exercises, you** movement, bench presses, inclined bench **risk having a fracture.** presses, cross cables, torso twisters or hip abductor/adductor movement in a semi-reclined position.

Yoga. A good yoga class should emphasize body alignment with special emphasis on the position of the back. Though many people are being instructed almost entirely in flexion movements, it is possible to do only the extension type movements. Discuss this with your yoga teacher.

Good yoga postures include the cobra, locust, boat, airplane, bridge, fish and bow, as well as any standing posture that emphasizes alignment of the back (mountain, tree, half moon, warrior and standing bow.)

T'ai chi. This ancient Chinese martial art employs slow, gentle dancelike movements. It can help improve balance, reaction time and strength, to reduce the risk of falls. If you decide to take t'ai chi classes, check to be sure your instructor is qualified.

> In one study, those who underwent t'ai chi training for 15 weeks reduced their risk of falling by 47.5% compared with those who didn't take the classes.

Stationary bicycle. Riding a stationary bicycle is not recommended. It is done in a seated position, which is the position of most spinal compression. A reclining bicycle would be better, as it places little stress on the spine. Adjust the bicycle's resistance to the lowest setting. Ride for 10 minutes twice a day during the first week, adding 1 to 5 minutes each week until you build up to 30-minute sessions. Then start gradually increasing the resistance.

Swimming. Swimming is not considered good exercise for osteoporosis because it is not weight bearing.

Water exercises. If you are too weak to walk far enough to make it worthwhile, starting out in the water can be helpful. Water therapy promotes flexibility and endurance and is fun to do, especially with a group. After water exercises and walking in water, you may be able to progress to walking and exercising out of the water.

Exercising in the water places less stress on your bones and joints than exercising on land. Plus, water assists in lifting your arms, so your muscles don't get as tired. Be careful not to overdo. Because the exercises seem so effortless, it is easy to overwork the muscles. If your muscles become stiff and sore, try over-the-counter analgesics, such as aspirin, acetaminophen or ibuprofen. A warm bath and a day or two of rest can also help relieve muscle pain.

Although it is unlikely that water exercises build bone, they can build muscles, improve balance and increase the range of motion in your joints, according to physical therapist Vibeke Vala. The following exercises can help strengthen your upper and lower back muscles. They are performed neck-deep in water. Begin with 1 to 5 repetitions, gradually working your way up to 10 or 15.

UNDERWATER LEG LIFTS: Stand in the pool with your feet slightly apart, your arms extended out at your sides. *Keeping your back straight,* swing your right leg upward about 45 degrees, then slowly return to the starting position. Repeat with the left leg.

THE BREAST STROKE: Extend your arms straight out in front of you with palms facing outward. Keep your elbows straight, and slowly swing your arms around your body and behind your back in a swimming motion. Bring your arms down to your sides, then return to the starting position.

SHOULDER PINCHES: Stand with your hands clasped (fingers interlaced) behind your back. Slowly roll your shoulders back as far as they will comfortably go and return to the starting position.

Site-specific exercises   Whether or not you have actually fractured, exercise is an essential part of your treatment. The pull of muscle on bone helps to strengthen the bone, and to be of most benefit, the exercise should be site-specific—in other words, exercise the muscle that attaches to the bone with depleted bone mass.

Because the primary problem with osteoporosis is compression and flexion (bending) of the vertebral column, exercises need to emphasize decompression and extension (straightening) movements.

Flexion exercises add to your risk of breaking a vertebra.

The ten exercises that follow are a sampling of exercises that can help when you have osteopososis. They are a good place to start and will give you a very good idea of what extension exercises feel like and how they can benefit you.

Follow these guidelines when you do the exercises:

• *Body position.* When lying on your back, there should not be a large space between your back and the floor; if there is, bend your knees so that your feet are flat on the floor and your lower back is as close to the floor as possible. That will relieve strain on your lower back.

You may need to support your head so it is not pushed too far forward or tilted back. Ask someone to help you by looking at your position.

If your shoulders are very high off the floor, place a support under them to even up the height of the shoulders with the head.

Place your arms slightly away from the body and turn your palms upward. Elbows should be at the same level as shoulders. If the elbows are lower than the shoulders, place support under them to make them level with the shoulders.

If you have an exaggerated curvature of the thoracic spine (dowager's hump), severely forward head, marked lumbar lordosis (swayback) and/or tightness of the muscles of the hip and thigh, you may have to support your head (if it is tilted back) and/or arms, and you may have to keep your knees bent until you get used to lying on your back.

Your goal is to be able to lie on your back with your knees straight and your head unsupported. Be patient. This may take several weeks or even months to accomplish, especially if you have not been able to lie on your back for several years.

• *Support.* Where you need to support a body part, use a small pillow or folded towel.

• *Where to exercise.* Exercise on the floor if you can, and lie on a mat or pad. If you have difficulty getting to and from the floor, use a bed in the beginning; but the bed will "give" and you will not obtain as much straightening of your back.

• *Number of repetitions.* When you are ready, start slowly, and gradually build in time and intensity. Generally, 3 to 8 repetitions of each exercise is sufficient, and more is not necessarily better. Fewer repetitions done correctly and completely are better than more of them done in a hasty, haphazard manner.

Fewer repetitions done correctly are better than more of them done haphazardly.

• *How often to exercise.* Make a commitment to do the exercises 1 or 2 times daily for 6 to 8 weeks; because they reverse poor postural habits that you have had for a long time, it would be ideal to do them 2 or 3 times daily in the beginning. By then, you should notice a significant difference in how you feel.

• *Soreness.* You may notice some soreness as you begin the program. This is natural and can be treated with warm showers and baths, moist heat, ice and massage as needed.

Look at the first exercise. Lying on your back may not seem like a bona fide exercise but it is! This is the position of least compression on the vertebral column. As an exercise it can help straighten the curves of the back and take the compression off the vertebral bodies. In many persons it alleviates pain and backache and frequently allows them to return to daily activities that had been previously given up.

An exercise to straighten the curves of the back and alleviate pain.

Other exercises to help strengthen the back are performed from this position. Done as instructed, they can safely restore body alignment.

1. DECOMPRESSION OF THE SPINE

Lie on your back with your knees bent, feet flat on the floor.

With arms slightly away from the body, turn your palms upward and allow shoulders to relax downward. (If you are very comfortable in this position, straighten your legs and lie with your legs straight.)

Stay in position while you do the next 5 exercises. (Begin with 1–5 minutes and work up to 30–45 minutes in this position.)

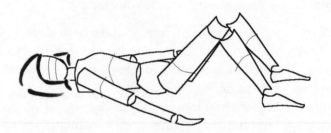

This position
- allows your vertebral column to straighten.
- takes compression off the vertebrae.
- is good to use when your back aches.

Remember, any floor exercise may be done on a bed if you have difficulty getting to and from the floor. But the bed will "give" and you will not obtain as much straightening of your back.

2. SHOULDER PRESS

Lie as in #1.

Press your shoulders back against the floor; hold for 3–5 seconds, then relax. (Knees may be bent to prevent arching of the lower back.)

Move only the shoulders—do not "hunch" your shoulders toward your ears and do not arch the lower back to get the shoulders down. Do not "roll" your arms.

If it is very difficult to do both shoulders at the same time, press one shoulder at a time and work up to being able to do both. The important thing to remember is to keep the motion all in the shoulders.

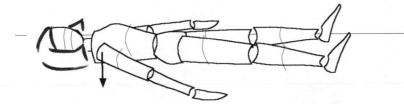

This exercise

• strengthens the muscles between the shoulder blades.

• strengthens the muscles that extend the spine and hold your back straight up against the force of gravity.

• stretches the muscles located on the front of the shoulder and chest.

3. CHIN TUCK

Lie as in #1.

Tuck your chin *SLIGHTLY* toward your chest and feel the lengthening of the back of your neck. (Knees may be bent.)

Holding the chin tucked (BUT DO NOT TILT YOUR HEAD BACK), press the back of your head back against the floor; hold for 3–5 seconds, then relax.

If the exercise is done properly, the entire head will move and slide slightly upon the floor. Do not try to tuck your chin by opening your mouth—the exercise is designed to re-align your HEAD position.

Touch the back of your neck lightly with your fingrtips and feel the muscles of the neck contract.

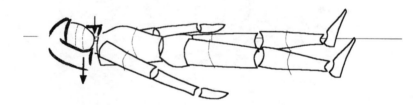

This exercise
- helps re-align the head over the shoulders.
- strengthens the muscles that hold the head up against the force of gravity.
- stretches the tight musculature on the front of the neck.

4. BUTTOCK SQUEEZE

Lie as in #1, with your hands in a comfortable position.

Extend your legs. (A small pillow may be placed under the knees to help reduce strain on the lower back.)

Squeeze your buttocks as tightly as possible (say "tight, tighter, tightest") and lift your tailbone slightly off the floor.

Hold for a count of 2–3 seconds, then relax.

Because this muscle group is weak in many people, you may have problems isolating it. Many people mistakenly do a pelvic tilt, contracting the abdominals rather than the buttock muscles.

To tighten the buttocks, it may help you to pretend that you have to go to the bathroom to have a bowel movement and you have to hold it; doing this will contract the correct muscle group.

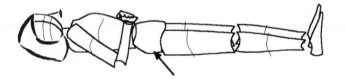

This exercise
- stretches the muscles located on the front of the hip.
- strengthens the buttocks and lower back musculature.

5. ARM LENGTHENER

Lie as in #1, with palms facing downward.

Keep your elbows straight, and bring one arm up and back alongside your head, trying to reach the wall behind you. (This pulls the rib cage up and away from the pelvis, and lengthens the space between the rib cage and hip.)

Hold for 3–5 seconds, then relax.

Repeat with other arm. (Or you can lengthen both arms together.)

As you do this exercise, contract abdominals and buttock muscles to prevent arching of lumbar spine.

Your lower back should remain flat against the floor. If it arches too much, keep your knees bent and feet flat on the floor.

The eventual goal is to be able to put your arms on the floor alongside your head. If you notice limitation of motion, go easy so you do not develop shoulder pain. If one arm is painful, it might help to hold a cane or stick in your hands and bring both arms up and back together; in that way, your stronger arm will assist and control the weaker, painful one.

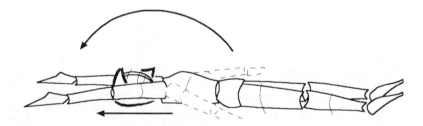

This exercise

• increases shoulder range of motion.

• stretches the muscles located along the sides of your body between the rib cage and pelvis.

6. LEG LENGTHENER

Lie as in #1.

Start with both knees bent.

Straighten one leg down to the floor; pull toes and forefoot up toward your knee.

Extend heel and "lengthen" leg by pulling your pelvis down away from the rib cage. *(The movement should occur primarily at waist level.)*

Hold position 2-3 seconds, then relax. Repeat with same leg.

Now do two "lengtheners" with the other leg.

Do in "sets" of two, for a total of 4–6 lengtheners on each leg.

If you have a lot of tightness when you pull to "lengthen" your leg, or if the movement triggers lower back discomfort, you may need to start more gradually. For each leg:

(1) Straighten leg down to floor, hold momentarily in the position, then rebend your knee;

(2) Straighten leg down again, pull toes and forefoot up, hold that position for 2-3 seconds, relax the foot, pull it up again, and re-bend the knee.

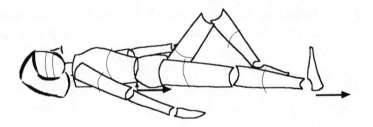

This exercise

• stretches the heelcord and calf musculature.

• stretches the muscles on the front of the hip joint.

• strengthens the buttocks muscles, the muscles on the front of the knee and the muscles that pick up your foot when you walk.

7. BELLY PRESS

Lie on your abdomen.

Rest your head on forehead or chin.

Place your hands underneath your prominent hip bones, and press your belly into the floor.

Hold 2–3 seconds and release.

You may notice some lifting of your legs and lower back as you press into the floor—do not try to move your legs or back, just press into the floor.

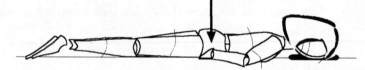

This exercise

 • strengthens the buttocks, upper hamstrings and lower back extensors (the muscles that straighten your back and help hold your body up against the force of gravity).

8. SHOULDER RETRACTION

Stand with good posture and lift chest slightly.

Interlace your fingers behind your back, keeping elbows straight. *If this is a strain for you, grasp a stick, cane or washcloth in your hands.*

Squeeze your backbone with your shoulder blades.

Hold 2–3 seconds and relax.

Do not thrust your head forward; do not "hunch" your shoulders toward your ears; do not arch your lower back or move your hands away from your body—the movement is all in the shoulders.

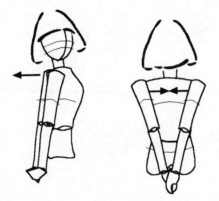

This exercise

- strengthens the muscles between the shoulder blades.
- stretches the muscles across the front of the shoulders and chest.

9. EXTENSION-IN-STANDING

Stand with your feet hip distance apart.

Place hands on waist with *thumbs facing forward*.

Squeeze buttocks together and press hips forward over the knees. *Do not arch your back or try to bring your shoulders back; this should be a gentle forward movement of the hips.*

Hold 2–3 seconds and relax.

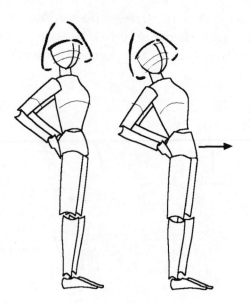

This exercise

  • strengthens the buttocks muscles.

  • stretches the muscles on the front of the hip joint, shoulders and chest.

  • is particularly good to do after being seated for a long time, such as on a long car ride or working at a desk or computer.

10. PUSHAWAYS

Stand facing a wall, corner or doorway.

Place hands on the wall at shoulder level.

Keep your body absolutely straight, elbows up, and lean into the wall.

Hold position for 3–5 seconds, then push away with your arms.

Your body should remain straight and your heels stay on the floor. If your heels come up, move closer to the wall so they stay on the floor. Think of this exercise as a push-up in a standing position.

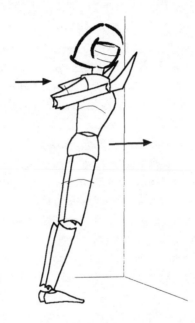

This exercise
- strengthens the muscles between the shoulder blades.
- strengthens the muscles of the arms.
- stretches the heel cords.
- stretches the muscles across the front of the shoulders and chest.
- is a good beginning weight-bearing exercise for the arms.

These exercises are part of a comprehensive program that includes posture, body mechanics, gait mechanics and balance. For more information, see page 238.

Case report: Valerie, age 74

*Valerie is a caucasian female who sustained compression frac-
tures of L1, L2, L3 and L4 while doing an "abdominal crunch"
exercise at a fitness center. Pain was immediate; she stopped exercising and sought medical attention.*

*The diagnosis of compression fracture was not made until
6 months later; during that time she was unable to obtain relief
of symptoms with medication. When the diagnosis was made,
a back brace was prescribed. She began physical therapy 4
months after that.*

*At the time of her initial physical therapy evaluation,
Valerie complained of mild back pain; she was still wearing
the brace and was afraid to do any exercise or even move for fear
of pain. Her score on the REEDCO (the posture test we use) was
67 (out of 100), with a moderate forward head posture, severely flattened lower back, moderately protruding abdomen,
moderate instabilility of both ankles, a moderate scoliosis,
slight tilt of her head and uneven shoulder height. Body height
was 5' 3" which represented a loss of about 1.5".*

*She was started on a $2^{1}/2$-month program of physical
therapy that included back strengthening exercises plus instruction in body mechanics, postural exercises and gait training.
During the course of treatment, she packed boxes in preparation
for moving in with her daughter. After packing, she experienced
severe pain and muscle spasms in the mid-back area. Medication
did not help her.*

*She returned to physical therapy, where she was treated
with moist heat and galvanic electrical stimulation to the involved area and instructed to continue with her exercises, body
positioning, body mechanics, and walking. Her symptoms were
relieved with two treatments.*

*At the time of discharge, Valerie was pain-free and on an
active exercise program, walking regularly. She had resumed
her normal lifestyle and no longer wore the back brace. Her
REEDCO posture score was 80 / 100, with improvements noted
in head position, shoulder height, head posture, abdomen pro-
trusion and lower back posture. She was instructed to avoid*

*any forward bending type of exercise, either at home or if she
should return to a fitness center.*

Case report: Grace, age 91

*Grace is a caucasian female who was referred to physical ther-
apy because of long-standing low back pain and severe thoracic
kyphosis (dowagers hump). She had given up hope of ever being
able to lead a normal life again and had resigned herself to a
wheelchair. She was in severe pain, was unable to stand for more
than 5 minutes and could barely get herself something to eat.
She lived alone and wanted to continue doing so as long as she
could.*

*At the time of her initial evaluation, her REEDCO posture
score was 35/100, with a deviation of her head to the right,
uneven shoulder height (left higher than right), severe scoliosis,
uneven hip height (right higher than left), moderate instability
of both ankles, severe forward head posture, severe thoracic kyphosis, moderately protruding abdomen and a flattened lower back.
She complained of severe low back pain and weakness and "ter-
rible leg cramps at night."*

*She had a long history of progressive spinal deformity and
compression fractures. Due to her severe pain and lack of
endurance, she was not put through the entire evaluative process.*

*Because of her frail condition and extensive postural dys-
function, Grace was seen for 41 total visits spaced one and two
weeks apart. She was fitted with a CASH orthosis (type of
brace) that allowed her to perform activities of daily living in
a more efficient manner. She was given exercises for strengthening, active isolated stretching, gait training, posture and
balance. Moist heat and electrical stimulation were used to relieve
pain and strengthen the back musculature.*

*At the time of discharge, Grace no longer had leg cramps,
and she was able to control back discomfort with body positioning, body mechanics, exercises and use of moist heat at home.
She became more active, driving her car to shop and to visit rel-
atives and friends, and visiting a fitness center for resistive exercises. She had also begun a daily walking program and followed*

a home exercise program with the help of an audio tape. She wore her brace daily but was able to go several hours a day without it.

Grace reported that she felt that she had a new lease on life because of the exercise program.

MEDICATION

Physicians can effectively treat most women with osteoporosis and keep them from sustaining more fractures. A key is early drug therapy and monitoring your response to therapy with bone density and appropriate lab testing.

Once you have lost a significant amount of bone mass, proper nutrition and exercise alone are not enough to reduce the risk of new fractures. When used in combination with drug therapy, however, they can enhance the beneficial effects of the drugs and may in fact reduce the dosages required.

The following medications may be prescribed to treat your osteoporosis. They are described more fully in Chapter 8.

Estrogen therapy is the most accepted means of managing established osteopososis, even if it was not used to prevent bone loss in the first place. If your uterus is intact it is imperative that you also take a *progestogen* to protect the uterine lining. Actually, a combination regimen can enhance the benefits of estrogen.

Fosamax is a new drug that can stop bone loss, build new bone as effectively as estrogen, and prevent hip, spine and wrist fractures. One pill is taken each morning with a glass of water, and then you must stand or sit upright and not eat anything for 30 minutes.

Calcitonin appears to help most when the problem is caused by increased calcium excretion. Calcitonin also has pain-relieving properties. It can be given either as an injection or as a nasal spray, which is more convenient.

Thiazide diuretics decrease the amount of calcium excreted in the urine and preserve bone density. Several studies have found that they reduce the risk of a hip fracture by up to one-third.

Tamoxifen inhibits bone breakdown and preserves bone mass. It is an established treatment for breast cancer that is not presently FDA-approved for treating osteoporosis.

Raloxifene is a close cousin of tamoxifen but has a better bone-mineral enhancing effect. Its efficacy is about half of that associated with estrogen use. Raloxifene appears to exhibit some of the positive effects of estrogen, including an antiresorptive effect in bone, and a cholesterol lowering effect.Unlike estrogen, it does not stimulate the uterine lining (endometrium), and it behaves as an anti-estrogen in breast tissue.

The following drugs have bone preserving properties. Before they can be approved for treating women with osteoporosis, however, there must be sufficient long-term studies on large groups of women to know how effective they are and what side effects can be expected.

Etidronate has been used successfully by doctors to increase bone mass and reduce spinal fractures. But it is not presently FDA-approved for treating osteoporosis.

Fluoride therapy builds bone but it has not been approved by the FDA to treat osteoporosis. Controversy still exists as to whether the newly formed bone is normal in composition. Some doctors believe that low-dose plain or slow-release fluoride in combination with estrogen, calcium and/or vitamin D will be effective in substantially increasing bone mass.

Risedronate has many of the benefits of Fosamax, perhaps without the gastrointestinal side effects.

PREVENTING FALLS

A fall that results in a broken hip is the leading cause of accidental death in elderly white women in this country. More than 90% of hip fractures occur after a fall. Falling can also cause other fractures, especially in the wrist.

What you can do. Think about and try to protect yourself from falling. In addition to practicing good body mechanics and increasing muscular strength and coordination, here are some other measures you can take.

1. Safeguard your house.

GENERAL: Move clutter or furniture away from where you walk. Make sure that electrical and telephone cords aren't stretched across walkways. If your bed has wheels, make sure they are locked. If the bed is high, consider getting a frame that's lower to the ground.

FLOORS: Avoid waxing floors, and be careful when floors are wet. Repair torn carpets; use tape to secure loose rugs Wear shoes or slippers with non-skid rubber soles. Do not walk around in your stocking feet.

LIGHTING: Keep your home well-lit, inside and out. Have light switches near the entrance of every room and near your bed, and make sure you can reach them easily. Place night lights throughout the house.

STAIRS: Make sure that stairs (outside porch stairs, too) have handrails and are well lit. Add nonskid treads on steps.

BATHROOM: Use a non-skid bathmat. Keep the floor dry. Install grab bars and a non-skid rubber mat in the bathtub or shower and near the toilet. Don't use bath oils; they can make the tub slippery. Consider a shower chair.

2. Look where you walk.
Take a little extra time to get where you're going. Move deliberately and carefully. Beware of curbs, uneven sidewalks, hard-to-see steps and other potential obstacles.

3. Have your vision and hearing checked annually.

4. Learn to manage postural hyoptension.
This is a dizziness and lightheadedness when you stand up quickly, caused by a sudden drop in blood pressure. Your physician can determine whether you have this problem by taking your blood pressure while you are seated and again while standing. If you have this problem, you need to:

- Get up slowly after sitting or lying down, and stand only when there is support to prevent you from falling.

- Wear elasticized support hose to help keep blood from pooling in your legs.

- Avoid alcohol, which can aggravate the condition.

- Avoid saunas, hot baths, steam baths and whirlpools, which lower blood pressure.

- Drink plenty of fluids, particularly in hot weather, when you have diarrhea or a stomach virus, or when flying on commercial airlines; all of these can cause you to become dehydrated, which will make the problem worse.

- Have someone elevate the head of your bed by stacking books or 2 x 6-inch blocks under the legs.

- Do these simple exercises before getting out of bed, to help raise blood pressure and circulate blood to your brain:

    (a) sit up with your feet hanging over the side of the bed, and flex your feet up toward you 5 or 6 times.

    (b) tense and relax your abdominal muscles several times.

    (c) tense the muscles in your hands and arms by making a fist several times.

Your physician may also recommend salt tablets or other medications. Salt tablets require medical supervision, since excessive sodium can *increase* blood pressure in some susceptible people.

5. Avoid alcohol, which can impair balance.

6. Have your back and musculoskeletal system examined. Your doctor can help assess the strength of your muscles and determine if you have very much disparity in leg length, which could cause you to lose your balance. You may need to strengthen your back and leg muscles and improve your posture.

7. Ask your doctor to assess your sense of balance. Tests may include standing on one foot, then placing heel of the other foot on the opposite knee; walking a straight line, one foot in front of the other;

standing still with eyes closed to see how much your body sways; with eyes closed, placing forefinger on nose.

8. Don't be vain; use a cane. Many women avoid using a cane or walker because they see them as symbols of disability and "old age." Remember: a little hurt pride heals a lot faster than a broken hip. Try to set aside your feelings and think of your physical health instead.

10. Ask your doctor about wearing a hip protector. An external hip protector acts as a shock absorber to help diffuse stress on the hip if you fall. They are made of polypropylene and plastic and are held in place by special underwear. The question is, how well do they actually protect?

> In a Danish study, 247 nursing home residents wearing a hip protector reduced their risk of hip fracture by 53%. Only 8 sustained a fracture, compared with 31 fractures in a comparison group.

> In laboratory studies at Beth Israel Hospital in Boston, Wilson Hayes, MD, found that many of the hip protectors presently available in the U.S. don't diffuse the force of a fall enough to prevent a fracture.

Research continues, and new products are being developed. You may wish to contact the National Osteoporosis Foundation for latest information as to what is available.

11. List all the medications you take and show it to your doctor. Sleeping pills, antidepressants and long-acting sedatives (causing drowsiness, confusion, dizziness and impaired coordination for 12 to 24 hours) can increase your risk of falling.

> A Vanderbilt University study found that women who take long-acting sedatives increase their risk of breaking a hip by 70%.

Ask your physician to review your medications and, where appropriate, switch to alternative drugs with a lower potential for side effects.

11 Osteoporosis in Men

This book is addressed primarily to women. But if you are a man, don't assume that you are immune from osteoporosis. Experts are just beginning to realize that osteoporosis is a significant and growing health problem for men as well.

About one-third of men will experience osteoporotic fractures during their lives. It may take you 20 to 30 years longer than a woman to lose enough bone to make you susceptible—men generally have bigger bones and more bone mass at skeletal maturity than women do—but whatever your age, osteoporosis can cause fractures, loss of height, pain and immobility, just as in women.

What are the causes? As with women, decline of bone mass begins in the mid-20s, with the loss of trabecular bone from the spine. Cortical bone mass reaches its peak around age 30 to 35, followed by a slight loss (.3 to .5% per year) until about age 50 (primarily from the long bones of the arms and legs). Like women, men then continue to lose bone slowly, but steadily, as a natural part of the aging process.

While many of the causes of osteopenia and fractures in men are similar to those in women, there are some notable differences.

Lack of testosterone (like lack of estrogen in postmenopausal women) is a factor, and although men do not experience menopause, they do have a gradual decline in reproductive hormones. Testosterone and other androgens begin to fall after age 35, and these hormones appear to be key factors for bone health.

- Androgens have been shown to have a direct effect on bone cells. Androgens increase production of the bone-forming osteoblasts (which have androgen receptors) and they change the way bone cells respond to parathyroid hormone (which stimulates bone-breakdown).

Androgen deficiency appears to be much more important to bone health than previously believed. Younger men with spinal fractures usually have had a longstanding testosterone deficiency. Many of the conditions leading up to bone loss, such as cancer, alcoholism and chronic illness, are associated with lower-than-normal testosterone levels. Low androgen levels can reduce vitamin D production, as can regular use of the drugs *diphenylhydantoin* and *phenobarbital*.

Who is at risk? Osteoporosis is especially likely in men who go through the "male menopause" and become sexually inactive. Other contributing factors are similar to those in women: chronic use of corticosteroids or thyroid hormone. Parathyroid hormone excess, particularly when coupled with lower-than-normal androgen levels (testosterone deficiency), places men at high risk.

Malnutrition and lack of dietary calcium and vitamin D also commonly contribute. Smoking, alcohol excess, arthritis, cancer, diabetes, thyroid and other hormonal problems may be additional factors. Men most likely to get osteoporosis have smaller bones and do not exercise regularly.

You should consider yourself at greatest risk if you have one or more of the following risk factors:

- Small stature and slender build
- Lower-than-average body weight
- Sedentary lifestyle
- Low-calcium diet
- Cigarette smoking
- Gastric surgery
- Chronic use of corticosteroids
- Heavy use of alcohol
- Rheumatoid arthritis, hyperthyroidism, hyper-parathyroidism, type I diabetes, chronic liver or kidney disease
- Regular and/or prolonged use of steroids, thyroid hormones, anticonvulsants, heparin, or chemotherapy
- Low testosterone levels

Of course, a bone density test is one of the most definitive ways to gauge whether or not you are at risk. We recommend that if you have one or more of the above risk factors you should consider having a test to determine whether you have low bone mass or are losing bone at a higher-than-expected rate.

Bone density tests should be accompanied by blood tests for bone-specific alkaline phosphatase and urine tests for the calcium-to-creatinine ratio and the collagen cross-link N-telopeptide (NTx) or deoxypyridinoline (D-PYR), all of which can help determine the rate of bone loss *(see Chapter 5)*.

If bone density and blood and urine tests reveal a problem, additional diagnostic tests can be conducted to determine the cause of the accelerated bone loss. These may include tests for testosterone levels and thyroid function. Reliable tests for parathyroid hormone and vitamin D are also available.

How can you prevent osteoporosis? You need to do everything you can to achieve high bone mass early in life. Exercise regularly and eat plenty of calcium-rich foods. Review your risk factors and have your bone density tested if you are at risk. If bone density is low, you can take measures to prevent further bone loss.

If you are at risk, consider taking many of the same preventive measures as women: consume adequate calcium and vitamin D, exercise, stop smoking, and limit alcohol to two drinks a day. You should also avoid excessive amounts of aluminum-containing antacids, and check with your doctor about making substitutions for any bone-dissolving medications you take.

Managing osteopenia and osteoporosis   For men with significant osteopenia or osteoporosis, adequate exercise, calcium and vitamin D are a must. Testosterone replacement therapy may be useful when testosterone levels are low. Treatment involves testosterone injections (if there is no prostate trouble). Consider also testosterone patches.

You should also respond well to treatment with antiresorptive drugs, such as bisphosphonates and calcitonin. Appropriate clinical trial data is not available, so consult with your physician regarding the relevance of these drugs to your situation. Also, ask about combining testosterone with a bisphosphonate drug.

If you have osteoporosis, the ten exercises in Chapter 10 can help strengthen your back and safely restore body alignment.

RECOMMENDED CALCIUM AND VITAMIN D FOR MEN		
AGE	CALCIUM (mg)	VITAMIN D
19–30	1,000	200 IU
31–50	1,000	400 IU
51–70	1,200	400 IU

Recommendations are based on best current information in published clinical resources and accepted medical practice, and incorporate the 1997 federal guidelines from the National Academy of Sciences..

12 Planning a Healthy Future

For the first time, fractures from osteoporosis may be almost entirely preventable. Scientists now understand what causes porous bones, they know what kinds of treatments can stop bone loss and strengthen the skeleton after bone mass has been lost, and, most important of all, *they know how to prevent the problem in the first place.*

The place to start is with a bone density test. The test lets you know whether your bone density is normal or if you are losing bone. With this information, the next step is obvious: either you do nothing (if density is normal) or, if density is low, you must take steps to stop bone loss and perhaps build new bone as soon as possible, before a weakened bone breaks.

In the past doctors depended on risk factors *(Chapter 4)* to decide who should be offered preventive therapy. But information from the medical and family history, including an assessment of lifestyle and other risk factors, identifies only about 30% of those

183

who have osteopenia. Now we can do better. Bone density testing (especially when combined with selective biochemical lab tests) can identify virtually 100% of those at risk. It can also track whether bone is being depleted and how your treatment is working.

Your doctor may not be aware of this lifesaving breakthrough! (Only 15 to 20% of women at risk currently receive preventive treatment.) *This is <u>your</u> body and <u>your</u> health, and you are going to have to take responsibility for it.* Don't wait until you have a symptom—the only symptom is a fracture. If you have any reason to think you are at risk, ask your doctor for a bone density test.

Preventive measures are always preferable to treatment, and prevention of osteoporosis should begin early. Physical activity in childhood is an important determinant of peak bone mass. Studies have shown that exercise habits started before the age of 10 continue throughout life. If you are a teenager or young adult, it may be difficult for you to imagine that today's poor nutrition, exercise and lifestyle habits could lead to disability in your later years. If you are menopausal, and you haven't already started a program of prevention, it's not too late to begin.

Many new therapies are being developed to halt bone loss and build bone mass. (Finally, money is being allocated to research into women's diseases.) In addition to new drugs, scientists are looking into the benefits of combining treatments that are known to be effective. As younger women become aware of osteoporosis and the ease with which it can be prevented, the need for treatment will be reduced.

Prevention isn't difficult: First, make sure that you have regular exercise and a diet with plenty of calcium and vitamin D. Second, check your bone density. By following these simple recommendations for preventing bone loss, you will be able to "stand tall" and lead a healthy, active life.

Case Reports

These are actual case histories from the records of the Women's Medical and Diagnostic Center in Gainesville, Florida. They have been included to illustrate the multitude of variables that can affect a woman's bone health and to show how each of these is taken into consideration in planning a woman's program of prevention or treatment.

A postmenopausal woman who has osteopenia, for example, may also be at risk of developing cardiovascular disease. A woman with a vaginal infection may be found upon examination and testing to have osteoporosis.

Keep in mind that there is no typical woman, no typical osteoporosis, and no typical treatment that can help everyone.

You may find parts of the situations described here that are similar to your own. Do not, however, apply their treatment to yourself. Rather, you should work closely with your physician to tailor a treatment program to suit your own needs.

The bone density given in these case reports has been measured with dual energy x-ray absorptiometry (DEXA) of the wrist, spine or hip. Results are given as a percentage of "peak bone mass," the average bone density of women at skeletal maturity.

WOMEN WITH NO SIGNS OF OSTEOPOROSIS

Mary, age 35

Mary's mother has osteoporosis, and Mary's concern that she, too, may be at risk of developing osteoporosis prompted her to take measures to keep her bones healthy and to have a bone density screening test of her wrist.

Mary's daily intake of calcium was 1,774 mg and vitamin D was an optimal 500 IU; she bicycled three times a week.

DEXA of wrist: 63%

Based on the low reading, she decided to have an evaluations of her hip and spine. They showed osteopenia.

DEXA of hip: 80%

DEXA of spine: 1st lumbar vertebra, 72%
    2nd, 3rd and 4th lumbar vertebrae, 78%

Mary continued to have adequate calcium and to exercise regularly, hoping that these measures would prevent further loss of bone mass. She was tested again the following year:

DEXA of hip: 80%

DEXA of spine: 1st lumbar vertebra, 67%

To help prevent further loss and possibly increase bone mass in her spine, we prescribed low-dose oral contraceptives. We encouraged Mary to keep up her calcium and vitamin D intake and her regular exercise program.

She will continue to have her bone density monitored for the next three to five years to make sure that these measures are helping. With this approach, we should be able to increase Mary's bone mass by the time she reaches menopause and prevent bone loss afterward.

Bonnie, age 38

Bonnie's uterus and ovaries were removed for the treatment of endometriosis when she was 37 years old. Afterward, she developed severe menopausal symptoms that were not relieved by Premarin, Estrace, Ogen, or the Estraderm patch.

Estrogen also gave Bonnie side effects: dizziness, headaches, nausea, and a general sense of malaise. When she stopped the estrogen, she experienced hot flashes, insomnia and fatigue. She also had vaginal dryness, which decreased her sexual desire.

Testing showed osteoporosis in both her spine and hip:

DEXA of spine: 2nd and 3rd lumbar vertebrae, 74%;
  4th lumbar vertebra, 65%

DEXA of hip: femoral neck 61%, Ward's triangle 49%

These values showed that Bonnie was at very high risk of sustaining a fracture.

We placed her on low-dose oral contraceptives (which had not produced side effects in the past) and soon afterward the menopausal symptoms subsided.

With her new regimen of oral contraceptives plus adequate calcium, a supervised exercise program and having her bone density monitored, Bonnie can anticipate a definite improvement in bone mass.

Paula, age 42

As part of a routine premenopausal evaluation, Paula had a bone density test of her wrist when she was still menstruating. She had none of the traditional risk factors for osteoporosis, and in addition, she was overweight (a protective factor).

DEXA of wrist: 78%

One year later the test was repeated:

DEXA of wrist: 75%

DEXA of spine: 1st lumbar vertebra, 77%;
  rest of spine, normal

We advised Paula to increase her calcium intake and begin a regular exercise program. Two years later:

DEXA of spine: 1st lumbar vertebra, 84%

And four years later:

DEXA of spine: 1st lumbar vertebra, 95%

During her most recent evaluation, five years after beginning her program of prevention:

DEXA of spine: 1st lumbar vertebra, 102%

Paula's case illustrates the point that lifestyle measures, such as regular exercise and adequate calcium, can make a dramatic improvement in the health of your bones, especially during your premenopausal years.

Suzanne, age 34

This story illustrates the importance of having a bone density test if you have a history of amenorrhea or irregular menstrual cycles.

Suzanne fractured her 2nd lumbar vertebra in a skiing accident and was referred to our clinic for an osteoporosis evaluation. Her calcium (2,000 mg/day) and vitamin D intake (500 IU) were more than adequate and she swam three times a week. We tested her bone density and found it was low.

DEXA of spine: 1st lumbar vertebra, 62%

DEXA of hip: Ward's triangle, 68%; femoral neck, 74%

Suzanne's medical history revealed the likely source of her problem: although she had started menstruating around age 13, her periods stopped a year later. She was not treated for the condition until she was 23 years old. With treatment she resumed normal periods.

When we saw Suzanne, her main dilemma was whether or not she should become pregnant again (she had one child). She also wondered if she should begin taking hormones or other medication used in the treatment of osteoporosis.

We advised her to become pregnant as soon as possible, both

because she was 34 years old (pregnancy-related risks rise with age) and because pregnancy could actually help increase bone density (provided she maintains adequate calcium intake). But we suggested that she breastfeed for only a short time, as breastfeeding encourages the loss of calcium from the skeleton.

We also advised her to begin weight-bearing and muscle-strengthening exercises, plus aerobic exercises such as treadmill, walking, riding a stationary bicycle, or using a Stairmaster.

As soon as she has weaned the baby, we will recommend that Suzanne go on low-dose oral contraceptives until she reaches menopause.

Gail, age 47

Gail came to the clinic seeking help for mood swings, night sweats and heart palpitations. Although she was still menstruating on a regular basis, her periods had become lighter and slightly more irregular over the past year. She also complained of vaginal dryness.

Gail's nutritional evaluation revealed that her calcium intake was almost nonexistent: just 177 mg per day, and she had virtually no vitamin D. She drank 10 cups of coffee and smoked half a pack of cigarettes a day. She did no exercise.

Her test results were not surprising.

DEXA of spine: 1st and 2nd lumbar vertebrae, 70%

DEXA of hip: Ward's triangle, 80%; femoral neck, 82%

Fortunately, Gail's problem was caught in plenty of time to do something before loss of bone mass was accelerated by approaching menopause. We advised her to increase calcium and vitamin D intake with high-calcium foods and supplements (1,000 mg of elemental calcium daily and a multivitamin), drink less coffee, and begin a regular exercise program that includes both muscle strengthening and aerobics. She was also advised to begin a non-oral form of estrogen, such as the skin patch, along with oral micronized progesterone (to be taken during the last 12 days of her menstrual cycle) to help protect her bones.

Betsey, age 58

Both of Betsey's sisters had breast cancer. For this reason, she was reluctant to take estrogen after her surgical menopause 11 years earlier. Instead, she made sure she had enough calcium (1,400 mg/day) and vitamin D. Since her occupation as a farm worker involved regular, heavy physical activity, she felt that she was getting plenty of exercise. She did not smoke, drink alcohol in excess, or consume excessive amounts of caffeine.

Betsey's main complaint when she came to the clinic was vaginal dryness—a consequence of her surgical menopause. However, routine bone density tests over the next two years revealed that she was losing bone in her hip at a rate of about 1% per year. Although the bone density of her spine actually increased during the same 2-year period, at 76% it was still low for a woman her age.

In spite of her family history of breast cancer, Betsey was advised to use a very low dose of Estrace estrogen cream vaginally for vaginal dryness. Because estrogen creams are absorbed into the bloodstream, Betsey's blood estrogen levels will be periodically monitored to ensure that they are not raised by the treatment.

To protect her bones, Betsey was offered either etidronate (alendronate was not available at the time) or calcitonin, and she was advised to take a thiazide diuretic to help increase the bone mineral content of her hip. We also encouraged her to begin a regular exercise program, since hard physical labor in itself is not necessarily protective.

Monica, age 62

Monica came to our clinic seeking treatment for hot flashes. Because she was menopausal, she consented to have her bone density tested. Although the bone mineral in her hip was adequate, her spine showed osteoporosis:

DEXA of spine: 2nd and 4th lumbar vertebrae, 74%
    1st lumbar vertebra 64%

She began hormone therapy (.625 mg of Premarin daily) for her hot flashes and to prevent further loss of bone mass in her spine.

Two years later, we persuaded her to have another bone density test (she didn't feel it was necessary because she was taking estrogen to protect her bones and she felt quite well).

DEXA of spine: 1st spinal vertebra, 58%

Based on this unexpected drop in bone mass, we tested Monica's blood levels of circulating estrogen. We found they were only about half as high as they should have been for the amount of estrogen she was taking. We increased her estrogen to .9 mg Premarin daily..

Monica will be monitored with blood and bone density tests to ensure that the treatment is working as it should. If blood estrogen levels don't rise, we will advise her to switch to a non-oral type of estrogen, such as a skin patch.

Grace, age 60

Postmenopausal women who can't take hormones can be treated with other medications that are known to stimulate new bone formation.

Grace experienced a natural menopause around age 52 and had never taken postmenopausal hormones because she had had two episodes of phlebitis (an inflammation of the wall of the leg veins)—once after giving birth to her second child and again about 10 years before visiting our clinic. The second episode of phlebitis occurred spontaneously along with a deep vein thrombosis (blood clot in the leg) that required hospitalization.

An osteoporosis evaluation revealed that Grace had a mild-to-moderate degree of osteopenia in her spine with osteoporosis in her hip.

DEXA of spine: 1st, 3rd and 4th lumbar vertebrae, 78%

DEXA of hip: Ward's triangle, 68%; femoral neck, 78%

Grace was treated with a short course of sodium fluoride (to stimulate new bone formation) together with a thiazide diuretic to improve the bone density of her hip. She was also encouraged to maintain a calcium intake of 1,400 mg per day.

One year later, the bone density in Grace's spine improved by 11%. The bone density in her hip increased by about 4%. She stopped the sodium fluoride and was placed on etidronate for two weeks every three months. She continued taking the thiazide diuretic. A year later, we again tested her bone density:

DEXA of spine: 93%

DEXA of hip: Ward's triangle, 79%; femoral neck, 89%

Grace will continue treatment for as long as it doesn't cause any serious side effects, and quite possibly for the rest of her life.

Marilyn, age 63

Marilyn, who was postmenopausal, came to the clinic seeking treatment for vaginal dryness. She had a family history of osteoporosis.

Because her natural menopause had come early, when she was only 45, we did a bone density test of her wrist on the first visit. Even though Marilyn was a lacto-ovo vegetarian, which some studies suggest may help protect against osteoporosis, the bone density of her wrist was low:

DEXA of wrist: 74%

We advised Marilyn to have a bone density evaluation of her hip and spine, but she decided not to do so at the time. A year later, when a repeat test of her wrist was found to be almost identical to the first—73%—she changed her mind.

DEXA of hip: Ward's triangle, 64%; femoral neck, 76%

Marilyn also had osteoporosis in her spine:

DEXA of spine: 2nd, 3rd and 4th lumbar vertebrae, 72%
    1st lumbar vertebra, 68%

Because she had a family history of breast cancer, Marilyn was reluctant to take estrogen. So we prescribed a low dose of estrogen cream for her vaginal dryness and advised her to have annual mammograms and to practice regular breast-self examination.

For her osteopenia, Marilyn began treatment with etidronate (alendronate would be used now). She was advised to increase her calcium intake from 720 to 1,400 mg per day.

With this program, Marilyn can expect to see a definite improvement in the bone density of her hip and spine over the next two to three years.

Kate, age 46

Kate came to the clinic complaining of recent poor memory and confusion. She had had a surgical menopause around age 25 for the treatment of growths on her ovaries; afterward she was placed on oral estrogen therapy, which she took for 20 years.

Kate's calcium intake was adequate at 1,400 mg per day, and her vitamin D intake was 400 IU. She exercised 2 to 3 times per week with both aerobic and muscle strengthening exercises. She did not smoke or drink caffeine-containing beverages, and only occasionally drank alcoholic beverages.

Bone density tests revealed that although she had been on hormone therapy and other measures to protect her bones for 20 years, Kate had a mixture of both osteopenia and osteoprosis:

DEXA of spine: 2nd, 3rd and 4th lumbar vertebrae, 77%
1st lumbar vertebra, 70%.

DEXA of hip: Ward's triangle, 73%; femoral neck, 79%

These values were very low for a woman Kate's age. To remedy the problems, we switched her to the Estraderm patch (we would now use Vivelle or Climara). Although her symptoms improved, blood tests revealed that not enough estrogen was getting into her bloodstream. In order to provide an adequate dosage of estrogen, Kate was advised to use the skin patch 3 times a week. If her blood estrogen levels do not improve, we will suggest that she switch to estrogen pellets.

WOMEN WHO HAVE OSTEOPOROSIS

Donna, age 64

Donna came to our clinic complaining of back pain, which prompted us to evaluate her for osteoporosis. Although she had been on hormone therapy after a natural menopause at age 45, she stopped nine years later because of breast tenderness.

An x-ray examination revealed two compression fractures in the 8th and 12th thoracic vertebrae.

DEXA of wrist (far distal radius): 49%

DEXA of arm (proximal radius): 58%

Subsequent bone density tests revealed that Donna had lost a considerable amount of bone in both her hip and spine:

DEXA of spine: 2nd, 3rd, and 4th lumbar vertebrae, 62%

DEXA of hip: Wards triangle, 36%; femoral neck, 62%

Treatment goals were to keep Donna from having more fractures by 1) preventing further bone loss with combination hormone therapy (estrogen and progestogen) and 2) increasing her bone mass with sodium fluoride therapy. She began a daily treatment regimen of estrogen, progestogen, and sodium fluoride. Donna was also advised to maintain her daily calcium and vitamin D intake at 1,500 mg and 400 IU, respectively.

Two years after beginning treatment:

DEXA of spine: 2nd, 3rd, and 4th lumbar vertebrae, 93%

DEXA of hip: Ward's triangle, 53%; femoral neck, 65%

Because of the great improvement, Donna stopped taking sodium fluoride; but she continued hormone therapy along with calcium and vitamin D.

Three years later, the bone density of her spine remained high:

DEXA of spine: 2nd, 3rd and 4th lumbar vertebrae, 92%

DEXA of hip: Ward's triangle, 66%; femoral neck, 77%.

What's more, she has not had any more fractures and is in excellent health.

Margaret, age 62

Margaret was diagnosed with breast cancer at age 49. Fortunately, the cancer was caught in its earliest stages and successfully treated with surgery. But because of her history of breast cancer, she decided not to take hormone therapy after a natural menopause at age 52. Ten years later, while visiting Europe, Margaret fell and fractured her pelvis.

After returning home, she came to the clinic for an osteoporosis screening and evaluation. We learned she had a family history of osteoporosis, she is lactose intolerant, she didn't exercise regularly, she smoked a pack of cigarettes a day, she was taking thyroid medication (Synthroid), her vitamin D intake was only 100 IU, and that her daily calcium intake was 342 mg—not even one-quarter of the recommended amount for women her age.

DEXA of spine: 2nd, 3rd and 4th lumbar vertebrae, 69%

DEXA of hip: femoral neck, 66%

TSH test: she was taking too much Synthroid.

To prevent further loss of bone mass and another fracture, we advised Margaret to start using the Estraderm skin patch. Even though she had had breast cancer, it had been 13 years since her surgery. Although a recurrence was possible with estrogen, the probability of a debilitating hip fracture in the near future was much greater.

With the skin patch we could easily monitor the levels of estrogen in her bloodstream to ensure that she didn't get too much. Margaret was instructed to examine her breasts once a week using breast self-examination, to have a breast exam by a health care professional every 6 months, and to have yearly mammograms.

If Margaret had chosen not to take estrogen, alternatives would have been etidronate or alendronate, and a thiazide diuretic together with a potassium supplement to counter potassium loss.

We advised Margaret to increase her calcium and vitamin D. Since she is lactose intolerant, we recommended either a calcium supplement or calcium-fortified orange juice. She was strongly encouraged to stop smoking and start exercising (brisk walking). We recommended that the Synthroid dosage be reduced and that she be monitored with TSH tests every three to six months.

Kimberly, age 57

Kimberly had a natural menopause when she was 52 years old and had been on hormone replacement therapy for several years. She stopped taking estrogen, however, when she heard reports that it may increase a woman's risk of breast cancer.

A year later, she fell and fractured her 3rd, 4th, 5th and 8th thoracic vertebrae. She came to the clinic with low back pain so severe that it interfered with her ability to perform even the simplest tasks. She had a family history of osteoporosis—her mother and grandmother had both suffered from it—that was compounded by her long-term use of Dilantin, which she took to control epileptic seizures.

Bone density evaluations revealed:

DEXA of spine: 2nd, 3rd and 4th lumbar vertebrae, 61%

DEXA of hip: Ward's triangle, 40%; femoral neck, 57%

If Kimberly fell during an epileptic seizure, her dangerously low bone mass put her at a very high risk fracturing her hip.

We convinced her that the benefits of estrogen—increased bone mineralization of the spine and, to a lesser extent, the hip, and protection from future fractures—far outweighed any possible increased risk of breast cancer. She decided once again to take combination hormone therapy, and when she was assessed six months later, the bone density of her spine had already improved by 4%.

Kimberly will be monitored closely over the next several years to ensure that the hormone therapy is working. She has also been advised to increase her calcium intake to 1,500 mg per day to help offset the effects of Dilantin on her bones, and to take every precaution against falling, which includes making sure that her seizures are well-controlled.

Carol, age 70

Carol had a natural menopause at age 51. Because she never had hot flashes or other symptoms of menopause, she did not take hormone therapy. Ten years later, she slipped in the bathtub and fractured a vertebra. The following month, she bent over and fractured another vertebra. She fractured a third vertebra a month later, when she fell over her bed. Some years later, she fractured a fourth vertebra when lifting a flower pot.

Four weeks prior to visiting our clinic, she developed severe back pain that was believed to be pleurisy, an inflammation of the delicate membrane covering the lungs. Subsequent examinations revealed, however, that the pain arose from wedging of two vertebrae, which occurred after Carol moved some furniture.

When she came to the clinic, Carol was taking .3 mg of Premarin, too small an amount to protect her bones. She was taking 3,400 mg of calcium, which far exceeded the recommended daily amount for women her age.

Carol had a marked reduction in bone mass:

DEXA of spine: 1st lumbar vertebra, 56%

DEXA of hip: Ward's triangle, 56%; femoral neck, 68%

We recommended that Carol increase her estrogen to .625 mg Premarin and also take a progestogen (2.5 mg of Provera) to protect against endometrial cancer and help increase bone mass. Since Carol's bone mass was dangerously low and she had already suffered a number of vertebral fractures, she was also advised to take sodium fluoride and a thiazide diuretic.

Two years after beginning treatment, the bone density of the 1st lumbar vertebra increased by 27%:

DEXA of spine: 1st lumbar vertebra 83%

The bone density of her hip had increased as well, although to a lesser extent:

DEXA of hip: Ward's triangle, 60%; femoral neck, 67%

Because her bone density had improved dramatically, Carol stopped taking fluoride, but continued hormone therapy and thiazide diuretics. A year later, bone density tests showed that the hormone therapy alone was preserving her bone mass. To further improve the bone density of her spine, we recommended increasing estrogen from .625 to .9 mg Premarin and her thiazide diuretic from 25 to 50 mg.

Since beginning treatment, Carol has been pain-free and has not had any further fractures.

Sarah, age 69

Sarah's story illustrates that it's never too late for hormone therapy. Sarah had a natural menopause at 50. When she came to the clinic at age 69, she had already had a series of vertebral fractures and was taking etidronate for 2 weeks every 2 months and 50,000 IU of vitamin D twice a week.

Sarah's bone density test indicated that she was at considerable risk of hip fracture.

DEXA of hip: Ward's triangle, 45%, femoral neck, 50%

DEXA of spine: 2nd, 3rd and 4th lumbar vertebrae, 51%

Sarah insisted on taking etidronate, but agreed to reduce her vitamin D. (Remember: too much vitamin D can actually stimulate bone loss.) A year later, she continued to lose bone and was persuaded to add a low dose of estrogen and a thiazide diuretic. At her next yearly examination, the bone density of her spine had improved somewhat, but she continued to lose bone in her hip:

DEXA of spine: 2nd, 3rd and 4th lumbar vertebrae, 57%

DEXA of hip: Ward's triangle, 26%

A urine test showed an increased calcium-to-creatinine ratio, indicating that Sarah was actively losing bone mineral. Based on these results, she was advised to increase her estrogen and the thiazide diuretic.

Another concern is that Sarah experiences occasional dizzy spells, which puts her at a much greater risk of falling and fracturing her hip. We gave her instructions on how to prevent falls and advised her to start a muscle strengthening exercise program, which should also improve her balance.

Leslie, age 59

Leslie came to the clinic because she had discomfort with intercourse as a result of vaginal dryness. She had had a natural menopause when she was 44 years old and had no other menopausal symptoms.

Leslie had a family history of diabetes (a brother and an aunt) and osteoporosis (maternal grandmother). She also had a weight problem: she was 5'7" tall and weighed 192 pounds. Although her weight would be expected to protect her against osteoporosis, an evaluation revealed that the bone density of her hip was markedly reduced.

DEXA of hip: Ward's triangle, 55%, femoral neck, 65%

Both of these values are substantially below average for her age and placed her at significant risk for hip fracture.

DEXA of spine: 79%

This is low, but still in the normal range for her age, illustrating that it is possible to have relatively normal bone density in the spine and low density in the hip. Also, that obesity does not exclude osteoporosis.

Blood cholesterol tests revealed that Leslie was at high risk of developing heart disease. This, added to her obesity and her family history of diabetes necessitated a treatment program that included dietary supervision and aerobic exercise for weight loss plus resistance exercise for osteoporosis. In addition, we prescribed continuous transdermal estrogen with natural progesterone of 200 mg/day for 12 days each month.

Given our policy of regular monitoring and adjusting dosage according to an individual's response, we can anticipate a healthy future for Leslie with a reduced risk of both heart disease and osteoporosis.

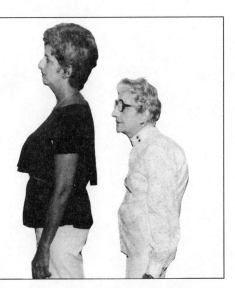

MOTHER AND DAUGHTER. The mother, age 76, has severe osteoporosis; she has lost 5 1/2" from her early adult height. Her daughter, age 56, has no outward signs of osteoporosis so far, but a bone density test indicates her bone mineral content is below average for women her age.

Glossary

ACUTE PHASE. The time immediately following fracture of a spinal vertebra, characterized by sharp pain at the level of the fracture.

ADRENAL GLANDS. Small, pyramid-shaped glands situated above the kidneys.

ADRENAL HORMONES. Substances manufactured and released by the adrenal glands. Some of these are harmful to bone.

ADRENOPAUSE. The time, usually around age 65, when the production of some of the adrenal hormones slows down.

AGONIST. Drug having an action similar to the natural compound.

ALKALINE PHOSPHATASE. Liver enzyme involved in calcium metabolism. Needs to be differentiated from bone specific alkaline phosphotase, a marker of new bone formation.

AMINO ACIDS. Organic compounds that are the primary components (building blocks) of proteins.

AMENORRHEA. Cessation of menstruation in a woman during the reproductive years.

ANABOLIC STEROIDS. Hormones that stimulate tissue growth; they are similar to the androgens.

ANDROGENS. Hormones responsible for the development and maintenance of male sex characteristics and reproductive function in men. Produced by the testes and adrenal glands in men, and by the adrenal glands and ovaries in women.

ANOREXIA. An eating disorder in which the affected person (usually a teenage girl or young adult woman), thinks she is "too fat," and eats so little that she literally starves. Associated with low body weight, cessation of menstruation, and loss of bone mass.

ANTACIDS. Preparations used to counteract overacidity in the stomach.

ANTICONVULSANTS. Drugs used to control seizures, as in epilepsy.

ANTIRESORPTIVE DRUGS. Drugs that slow down or stop bone loss, generally do not increase new bone formation. Examples: estrogen, calcitonin, alendronate (Fosamax).

APPENDICULAR SKELETON. Long bones of the arms and legs.

ARTHRITIS. Medical condition characterized by pain and inflammation of the joints. Two major types: osteoarthritis, rheumatoid arthritis. The latter is associated with low bone mass.

BICONCAVE. Having a depressed, or hollowed-out surface on both the upper and lower surfaces of a vertebra.

BISPHOSPHONATES. A class of drugs that is being investigated for the treatment of osteopenia and osteoporosis. Alendronate (Fosamax) is FDA approved.

BMD. Bone mineral density. Same as bone density, below.

BONE DENSITY. Measurement of the amount of bone mineral (mainly calcium) in tested areas of the skeleton. Result reported as GM/CM^2 (grams per centimeter squared).

BONE GLA PROTEIN. A peptide produced by the bone-building osteoblasts. Can be measured in blood and may serve as a useful marker of new bone formation.

BONE MASS. Total amount of bone mineral in the body. Increases from birth, reaching a peak around the age of 30. Thereafter, it declines as bone is lost with age.

BONE MINERALIZATION. Last step in the formation of new bone, when calcium and phosphorus crystals attach to the collagen matrix.

BONE REMODELING. Cyclic process of bone breakdown and formation that controls growth, maintenance, and repair of bone tissue.

BONE RESORPTION: Removal of "old" bone by cells known as osteoclasts.

BULIMIA. An eating disorder characterized by the consumption of unusually large quantities of food, followed by self-induced vomiting or use of laxatives to "purge" the food from the body. Associated with menstrual irregularities and low bone mass.

CALCITONIN. A "calcium-sparing" hormone released primarily by the thyroid gland. Acts to slow down bone breakdown. An injectible and nasal spray form of salmon calcitonin is used for treating osteoporosis.

CA-125. Substance produced by ovarian cancers, endometriosis, and uterine fibroids. Can be detected in blood, and is used in screening for ovarian cancer in women with suspicious pelvic masses.

CALCIUM. Metallic element found in nearly all living tissue. Gives bone most of its structural properties (99% of the body's calcium is in the bones) and is necessary for muscle contraction, blood clotting, and nerve impulse transmission.

CALCIUM BALANCE. The net of the processes in which calcium enters the body through the diet and leaves through sweat, urine, and feces. Negative calcium balance means that more calcium is excreted than taken in; positive calcium balance means more calcium is taken in than excreted.

CALCIUM "THERMOSTAT." Regulating mechanism that maintains a relatively constant level of calcium in the blood; involves parathyroid hormone, vitamin D, and calcitonin.

CALCIUM-TO-MAGNESIUM RATIO. Amount of calcium in the diet relative to the amount of magnesium in the diet.

CALCIUM-TO-PHOSPHORUS RATIO. Amount of calcium in the diet relative to the amount of phosphorus in the diet.

CALCITRIOL. An activated form of vitamin D in pill form that is selectively used as a treatment for osteoporosis in some countries, e.g., Japan. Not FDA approved yet.

CALIPERS. Instrument with two curved legs that can be adjusted to make fine measurements of thickness or width.

CASH ORTHOSIS. Trade name of a custom fitted brace that helps support the back and prevent forward besnding movements.

CAT (COMPUTERIZED AXIAL TOMOGRAPHY) SCAN. Same as CT scan.

CERVIX. Narrow lower end of the uterus that extends into the vagina. (Pap smears are taken from the cervix.)

CHRONIC PHASE. Period following the acute phase of a spinal vertebral fracture; characterized by a dull muscle ache in the mid or lower back.

CODFISHING. Refers to the fish-shaped appearance of the space between two adjacent spinal vertebrae, prior to their collapse.

COLLAGEN. Protein that is the supportive component of bone, connective tissue, cartilage, and skin.

COLLES' FRACTURE. Break in the lower part of the radius; commonly called a wrist fracture.

CORTICAL BONE. Hard dense layer that forms the outer shell of all bones.

CORTICOSTEROIDS. Drugs that resemble adrenal hormones; sometimes used to treat asthma or arthritis.

CORTISONE. An adrenal hormone that can be harmful to bone. Also refers to a drug resembling the adrenal hormone.

CROWN-TO-RUMP HEIGHT. A person's height from the top of the head to the bottom of the spine; method of monitoring height loss.

CRUSH or COMPRESSION FRACTURE. Spinal (vertebral) break in which both the upper and lower surfaces of the bone have collapsed.

CT SCAN. A method of viewing cross sections of tissue or bone with computer generated and controlled x-rays. (Same as CAT scan.)

CURETTE. Small instrument used to scrape portions of tissue from the lining of the uterus for later inspection under a microscope.

CUSHING'S SYNDROME. Overactivity of the adrenal glands.

DENSITOMETER. Instrument that measures bone density by determining the amount of radiation absorbed.

DIABETES. Disease that impairs the body's ability to use sugar. Two types: type I, insulin-dependent diabetes, has been associated with an increased risk of osteoporosis; type II, non-insulin-dependent diabetes, appears to have a protective effect.

DIURETICS. Drugs that promote the excretion of urine.

DIVERTICULITIS. Inflammation of the left side of the large colon; usually causes crampy pain in the lower left side of the abdomen.

DOWAGER'S HUMP. Protruberance of the upper back caused by collapsing of vertebrae and outward curvature of upper spine.

DUAL ENERGY X-RAY ABSORPTIOMETRY. Method of measuring bone density of the spine, hip, and wrist with x-ray radiation.

DUAL PHOTON ABSORPTIOMETRY. Method of measuring bone density of the spine and hip with gamma rays from a radioactive isotope (gadolinium).

ENDOMETRIAL BIOPSY. Removing a sample of the lining of the uterus for testing; also refers to the test itself.

ENDOMETRIAL CANCER. Cancer of the lining of the uterus.

ENDOMETRIOSIS. A sometimes painful condition in which endometrial tissue is found outside the uterus attached to the surface of the uterus, ovaries, tubes, rectum, or lining of the abdominal cavity (peritoneum).

ENDOMETRIUM. The lining of the uterus.

ENVELOPES. The lining of the surfaces of bone. The periosteal envelope is the outer surface, the endosteal envelope is the inner surface that lines the bone marrow cavity, and the intracortical envelope is the area between the two.

ERT. See Estrogen replacement therapy.

ESTROGEN REPLACEMENT THERAPY (ERT). Treatment to restore estrogen lost by removal of the ovaries (as after a surgical menopause) or to correct a hormonal imbalance or deficiency (as can occur after a natural menopause). See also hormone replacement therapy.

ESTROGENS. Hormones responsible for the development and maintenance of sex characteristics and reproductive function in women. Produced by the ovaries and fatty tissue in women. Also in small amounts by the testes in men. Pharmaceutical estrogens can be administered to women to correct hormonal problems.

FEMUR. Thigh bone (the longest and strongest bone in the body).

FEMORAL NECK. Narrow area at the upper part of the thigh bone.

FLUORIDE. Chemical element that promotes formation and growth of teeth and bones. Sometimes added to community water supplies to prevent dental cavities. Selectively used in the treatment of osteoporosis. Slow-release form of sodium fluoride has not yet been approved by the FDA for treating women with osteoporosis.

FOLLICLE STIMULATING HORMONE. Pituitary hormone that helps regulate the menstrual cycle. A blood test for FSH can help determine whether a woman is menopausal and whether postmenopausal estrogens are being properly absorbed and used by the body.

FRATERNAL TWINS. Twins that develop from separate fertilized eggs.

GnRH AGONISTS. Drugs that indirectly reduce estrogen and progesterone levels in the body, medically inducing a reversible menopause. Used for treating such gynecological problems as endometriosis, noncancerous fibroid tumors of the uterus, and severe premenstrual syndrome. If taken without estrogen for more than six months, the drugs can cause bone loss.

GROWTH FACTORS. Substances produced by bone and other tissues in the body; responsible for tissue repair and regeneration.

GROWTH HORMONE. Substance produced by the pituitary gland; stimulates growth in many tissues throughout the body.

HORMONE. A chemical substance produced in the body; when carried in the blood to another location it has specific effects.

HORMONE REPLACEMENT THERAPY (HRT). Treatment to correct a hormonal imbalance or deficiency (as can occur after a natural menopause) or restore hormones lost by removal of the ovaries (as after a surgical menopause). See also estrogen replacement therapy.

HRT. See Hormone replacement therapy.

HYPERCALCEMIA. Excess amounts of calcium in the blood.

HYPERPARATHYROIDISM. Overactivity of the parathyroid glands.

HYPERPROLACTINEMIA. Medical condition characterized by higher-than-normal blood levels of the breast-milk-producing hormone prolactin. Associated with cessation of menstruation, low estrogen levels, and bone loss.

HYPERTENSION. High blood pressure.

HYPERTHYROIDISM. Overactivity of the thyroid gland.

HYSTERECTOMY. Surgical removal of the uterus. Total or complete hysterectomy: surgical removal of both the uterus and cervix.

IDENTICAL TWINS. Twins that develop from a single fertilized egg.

KYPHOSIS. Outward curvature of the upper spine.

LACTASE. An intestinal enzyme that breaks down lactose, a sugar, into small, easily digested components.

LACTASE DEFICIENCY. Deficiency of the enzyme lactase, resulting in uncomfortable gastrointestinal symptoms when foods containing lactose are eaten. (Also called lactose intolerance.)

LACTATION. Breastfeeding.

LACTOSE. A sugar found in milk and other dairy products.

LACTOSE INTOLERANCE. Deficiency of the enzyme lactase, resulting in uncomfortable gastrointestinal symptoms when foods containing lactose are eaten. (Also called lactase deficiency.)

LORDOSIS. Inward curvature of the lower spine.

LUMBAR VERTEBRAE. Bones of the spinal column in the lower part of the back.

MENARCHE. Onset of menstruation during puberty; the first menstrual period. Begins for most girls between ages 12 and 16.

MENOPAUSE. Developmental phase characterized by decreased estrogen and progesterone production, the end of menstruation, and loss of child-bearing potential. Usually occurs around the age of 50.

METACARPALS. Bones of the hand between the wrist and fingers.

MICROFRACTURES. Fractures of the trabeculae in bone; these can only be demonstrated in biopsy samples of bone that have been magnified for viewing under a microscope. Microfractures do not cause symptoms, e.g., pain.

OOPHORECTOMY. Surgical removal of the ovaries.

OPAQUE SKIN. Skin of normal thickness, lacking transparency.

OSTEOBLASTS. Small cells that fill in the cavities "dug" by osteoclasts, producing the collagen matrix of new bone.

OSTEOCLASTS. Large cells that initiate the bone remodeling cycle by "digging" cavities in existing bone tissue.

OSTEOCYTES. Mature osteoblasts embedded in newly-mineralized bone.

OSTEOMALACIA. Bone disease in adults caused by vitamin D deficiency; characterized by inadequate mineralization of new bone. Results in "softer" bone.

OSTEOMARK. New, very sensitive urine test that specifically measures bone-specific collagen; can be used to assess efficacy of anti-resorptive drugs, e.g., estrogen, calcitonin and biphosphonates.

OSTEOPENIA. Reduction in overall bone mass to a level below "normal" but still above that associated with fracturing. Now defined as 10% (1 standard deviation) to 25% (2.5 standard deviations) below peak adult bone mass.

OSTEOPOROSIS. Reduction in overall bone mass (characterized by increased porosity and thinning of the bone) to the point that microscopic or more obvious fracturing has occurred. Also, bone density more than 25% below peak adult bone mass.

Primary osteoporosis cannot be traced to one single cause and is usually the result of interaction among genetic, nutritional, and environmental factors.

Secondary osteoporosis is usually the result of a drug or disease that causes bone loss.

Postmenopausal osteoporosis is directly related to the loss of estrogens and progesterone as well as to interactions of genetic, nutritional, and environmental factors.

Disuse osteoporosis is caused by prolonged immobilization, bed rest, paralysis, or weightlessness.

OXALATES. Compounds that can interfere with the absorption of calcium; found in some leafy green vegetables.

PARATHYROID GLANDS. Four tiny organs near the thyroid gland (two on each side) in the neck.

PARATHYROID HORMONE. Substance released by the parathyroid glands in response to low levels of calcium in the blood; stimulates bone breakdown in order to release calcium and restore normal levels in the blood.

PEAK BONE MASS. Values above 90% of the average bone density in a large population of "young normal women" at 35, the age when women reach skeletal maturity.

PELVIC INFLAMMATORY DISEASE. Bacterial infection of the lower pelvic region.

PERIODONTAL DISEASE. An inflammation of the gums; leads to loss of jaw bone, and loosening and sometimes loss of teeth.

PHOSPHORUS. Nonmetallic element found in all living tissues and involved in almost every metabolic process; provides (with calcium) much of the structural framework of bones.

PHYTATES. Compounds that can interfere with calcium absorption; found in the outer husk of cereal grains.

PITUITARY GLAND. Small oval organ at the base of the brain; called the "master gland," it produces many important hormones.

PLACEBO. An inactive substance, frequently in the form of a pill, used in controlled scientific studies to determine the effectiveness of drugs. Sometimes called a "sugar pill."

PLAQUE. Buildup of material on the teeth that can foster bacterial growth.

POSTURAL HYPOTENSION. Medical condition characterized by a sudden drop in blood pressure when a person sits or stands up quickly; can cause dizziness, lightheadedness, and sometimes fainting, all of which increase the risk of falling and fracturing a hip.

PROGESTERONE. Hormone produced by the ovaries during the second half of the menstrual cycle; acts to prepare the uterus for pregnancy.

PROGESTOGEN or PROGESTIN. Synthetic preparation that resembles the natural hormone progesterone.

PROLACTIN. Pituitary hormone involved in breast milk production.

PROSTAGLANDINS. Substances produced in bone and other tissues, such as the brain, breasts, blood vessels, and kidneys. In bone, prostaglandins are thought to help regulate the formation of new bone tissue.

PYORRHEA. Synonym for periodontal disease.

PYRILINKS D. New, very sensitive urine test that specifically measures bone-specific collagen; can be used to assess efficacy of anti-resorptive drugs, e.g., estrogen, calcitonin and biphosphonates.

RADIOGRAMMETRY. X-ray method of measuring the thickness of the outer cortical shell of bones.

RADIOGRAPHIC PHOTODENSITOMETRY. X-ray method of measuring the density of bones.

RADIUS. The smaller and shorter of the two bones of the forearm.

RECEPTOR. Tiny area on the surface of cells or membranes to which specific substances (e.g., hormones) "fit" (like a lock and key) and exert their biologic effects.

REEDCO POSTURE SCORE. Measuring tool used by physical therapists; based on observation of 10 aspects of standing posture. Perfect score is 100.

REMISSION. The time after a spinal vertebral fracture when symptoms and pain have abated; follows acute and chronic phases.

RESORPTION. Bone breakdown; part of the bone remodeling process.

RHEUMATOID ARTHRITIS. Chronic inflammatory disease of joints.

RICKETS. Bone disease of infants and young children caused by vitamin D deficiency; results in defective bone growth.

SEDIMENTATION RATE (SED RATE). Blood test used to help identify bone loss associated with a serious illness.

SINGLE PHOTON ABSORPTIOMETRY. Method of measuring the density of bone in the long bones of the body, usually the arm, using gamma rays.

SINGLE PHOTON X-RAY ABSORPTIOMETRY. Method of measuring the density of bone in the long bones of the body, usually the arm, using x-rays.

SURGICAL MENOPAUSE. Premature menopause brought on by surgical removal of the ovaries before a woman's natural menopause.

TAMOXIFEN. Drug commonly used in the treatment of breast cancer. Because tamoxifen has been found to enhance the effects of estrogen on bone, it may also be useful in the treatment of osteoporosis.

THIAZIDE DIURETICS. Drugs used to treat high blood pressure. Because they increase the reabsorption of calcium by the kidney into the blood system, may also help preserve bone mass.

THORACIC VERTEBRAE. Bones of the spinal column in the area of the middle of the back.

THYROID GLAND. Organ at the base of the neck primarily responsible for regulating the rate of metabolism.

THYROID HORMONES. Substances released by the thyroid gland that regulate metabolism; excessive amounts can cause bone loss.

TRABECULAR BONE. Porous, spongy bone that lines the bone marrow cavity and is surrounded by cortical bone.

TRANSPARENT SKIN. Thin skin through which the fine details of the underlying veins can be seen.

ULTRASOUND. High frequency sound waves used to measure the strength of bone, and probably indicative of the collagen content of bone and possibly its microarchitecture.

ULNA. The inner, larger bone of the forearm.

URINARY HYDROXYPROLINE. Urine test that reflects the breakdown of collagen in bone. Replaced by Osteomark and Pyrilinks D.

UTERUS. The womb.

VITAMIN D. Considered to be both a vitamin and a hormone; produced in the skin during sun exposure and available from several foods. In the body, vitamin D is one of the three hormones of the calcium "thermostat." Normal levels are beneficial to bone and promote calcium absorption and limit calcium excretion. High levels can cause bone loss.

VITAMIN K. Fat-soluble vitamin found chiefly in leafy green vegetables. Believed to play an important role in bone matrix formation and mineralization.

WARD'S TRIANGLE. Area on the uppor portion of the thigh bone where the main shaft of the bone is connected to the femoral neck. A common site for bone density tests of the hip.

WEDGE FRACTURE. Spinal vertebral break in which the front, but not the back, section of the vertebra has collapsed.

Bibliography

CHAPTER 1

Aaron FE et al. Osteomalacia and osteoporosis in fractures of the proximal femur. *Lancet* 1974; 1:299

Cooper C, Baker D. Risk factors for hip fracture. *N Engl J Med* 1995; 23:814-15.

Cummings S et al. Risk factors for hip fracture in white women. *N Engl J Med* 1994; 23:767-73.

Gallagher J C et al. Epidemiology of fractures of the proximal femur in Rochester, Minnesota. *Clin Ortho Rel Res* 1980; 149:207.

Hansen M et al. Spontaneous postmenopausal bone loss in different skeletal areas—followed up for 15 years. *J Bone Miner Res* 1995; 10(2): 205-10.

Heaney, R. Pathophysiology of osteoporosis. *Am J Med Sci* 1996; 312(6): 251-256.

Horsman A et al. Cortical and trabecular osteoporosis and their relation to fractures in the elderly. In *Osteoporosis: Recent advances in pathogenesis and treatment*, eds. H. F. DeLuca, et al. Baltimore, Maryland: University Park Press, 1981.

Iskrant AP. The etiology of fractured hips in females. *Am J Pub Health* 1968; 58:485.

Keene JS, Anderson CA. Hip fractures in the elderly. Discharge predictions with a functional rating scale. *JAMA* 1982; 248:564.

Knowelden J et al. Incidence of fractures in persons over 35 years of age. *Br J Prev Soc Med* 1974; 18:130.

McKenzie L, Notelovitz M. Osteoporosis-related fractures of the femur: The financial cost. Professional Communications, Inc: 1982.

Miller CW. Survival and ambulation following hip fracture. *J Bone Joint Surg* 1978; 60A:930.

Newton-John HF et al. The loss of bone with age, osteoporosis and fractures. *Clin Ortho Rel Res* 1970; 71:299.

Owen RA et al. The national cost of acute care of hip fractures associated with osteoporosis. *Clin Ortho Rel Res 1980;* 150:172.

Stewart IM. Fractures of the neck and femur: survival and contralateral fracture. *Br Med J* 1957; 2:922.

CHAPTER 2

Buchanan JR et al. Early vertebral trabecular bone loss in normal premenopausal women. *J Bone Miner Res* 1988; 3(5):583-587.

Dempster D, Lindsay R. Pathogenesis of osteoporosis. *Lancet* 341:797-806, March 1993.

Frost HM. *Bone remodeling and its relationship to metabolic bone diseases.* Springfield, Illinois: Charles C. Thomas, 1973.

Frost HM. Tetracycline-based histological analysis of bone remodeling. *Calcified Tissue Research* 1969; 3:211.

Gain SM. The phenomena of bone formation and bone loss. In *Osteoporosis. Recent advances in pathogenesis and treatment*, eds. HF Deluca et al. Baltimore, MD: University Park Press, 1981

Looker AC et al. Prevalence of low femoral bone density in older U.S. women from NHANES III. *J Bone Miner Res* 1995; 10(5):796-802.

Manolagas S, Jilka R. Bone marrow, cytokines, and bone remodeling. *N Engl J Med* 1995; 2:305-11.

Mazess RB. On aging bone loss. *Clinic Orth Rel Res* 1982; 165:239.

Notelovitz M. Osteoporosis: screening, prevention, and management. *Fertil Steril* Apr 1993; 59(4):707-725.

Riggs BL et al. Differential changes in bone mineral density of the appendicular and axial skeleton with aging. *J Clin Invest* 1981;67:328.

Riggs BL et al. Rates of bone loss in the appendicular and axial skeletons of women. *J Clin Invest* 1986; 77: 1487-1491.

Teegarden D et al. Peak bone mass in young women. *J Bone Miner Res* 1995; 10(5):711-715.

CHAPTER 3

Atkins D et al. The effect of oestrogens in the response to bone to parathyroid hormone in vitro. *J Endocrin* 1972; 54:107.

Boot, AM et al. Bone mineral density in children and adolescents: relation to puberty, calcium intake, and physical activity. *J Clin Endocrinol Metab* 1997; 82:57-62.

Brighton CT et al. *Electrical properties of bone and cartilage.* New York: Grune & Stratton, 1979.

Chen TL, Feldman D. Distinction between alpha-fetoprotein and intracellular estrogen receptors. Evidence against the presence of estradiol receptors in rat bone. *Endocrinology* 1978; 102: 236.

Chen TL et al. Glucocorticoid receptors and inhibition of bone cell growth in primary culture. *Endocrinology* 1977; 100:619.

Gallagher JC et al. Intestinal calcium and serum vitamin D metabolites in normal subjects and osteoporotic patients. Effect of age and dietary calcium. *J Clin Invest* 1979; 64:729.

Heath H, Sizemore GW. Plasma calcitonin in normal man. *J Clin Invest* 1977; 60:1135.

Jassal S et al. Low bioavailable testosterone levels predict future height loss in postmenopausal women. *J Bone Miner Res* 1995; 10(4):650-54.

Lloyd T et al. The effect of calcium supplementation and Tanner stage on bone density, content and area in teenage women. *Osteoporosis Int* 1996;6:276-283.

Matkovic, V. Nutrition, genetics, and skeletal development. *J Am Coll Nutr* 1996;15:556-569.

Meema S, Meema HE. Menopausal bone loss and estrogen replacement. *Isr J Med Sci 1976;* 12:9

Milhaud G et al. Deficiency of calcitonin in age-related osteoporosis. *Biomedicine* 1978; 29:272.

Orimo H et al. Increased sensitivity of bone to parathyroid hormone in ovariectomized rats. *Endocrinology* 1972; 90:760.

Prior JC. Progesterone as a bone-trophic hormone. *Endocrine Rev* 1990; 11(2):386-398.

Rico H et al. The role of growth hormone in the pathogenesis of postmenopausal osteoporosis. *Arch Int Med* 1979; 139:1263.

Shamonki IM et al. Age-related changes of calcitonin secretion in females. *J Clin Endocrin Metab* 1980; 50:437.

Stevenson JC et al. Calcitonin and the calcium-regulating hormones in postmenopausal women: effect of oestrogens. *Lancet* 1981; 1:693.

Tanaka Y et al. Sex hormone control of the renal vitamin D hydroxylases. In *Vitamin D: Biochemical, chemical and clinical aspects related to calcium metabolism*, eds. A.W. Norman, et al. New York: Walter de Groyter, 1977.

CHAPTER 4

Adachi, J. Corticosteroid-induced osteoporosis. *Am J Med Sci* 1997; 313(1):41-49.

Adland-Davenport P et al. Thiazide diuretics and bone mineral content in postmenopausal women. *Am J Obstet Gynecol* 1985; 152(6):630-634.

Bachmann GA. Hysterectomy: a critical review. *J Reprod Med* 1990; 35(9):839-861.

Barrett-Connor E, Holbrook TL. Sex differences in osteoporosis in older adults with non-insulin-dependent diabetes mellitus. *JAMA* 1992; 268(23): 3333-3337.

Bauer RL et al. Low risk of vertebral fracture in Mexican American women. *Arch Int Med* 1987; 147:1437-1439.

Bernstein DS et al. Prevalence of osteoporosis in high-and low-fluoride areas in North Dakota. *JAMA* 1966; 198:499.

Bones in Space. Editorial. *Br Med J 1980;* 1:1288.

Cann CE et al. Decreased spinal mineral content in amenorrheic women. *JAMA* 1984; 251(5): 626-629.

Chan GM et al. Bone mineral status of lactating mothers of different ages. *Am J Obstet Gynecol* 1982; 144(4):438-441.

Chestnut, CH et al. Hormone replacement therapy in postmenopausal women: urinary N-telopeptide of type I collagen monitors therapeutic effect and predicts response of bone mineral density. *Am J Med* 1997; 102:29-37.

Coindre JM et al. Bone loss in hypothyroidism with hormone replacement. *Arch Int Med* 1986; 146:48-53.

Cook B et al. An osteoporosis patient education and screening program: results and implications. *Patient Ed Counseling* 1991; 17:135-145.

Daniell HW. Osteoporosis and smoking. *JAMA* 1972; 221:509.

Daniell HW. Osteoporosis of the slender smoker: vertebral compression fractures and loss of metacarpal cortex in relation to postmenopausal cigarette smoking and lack of obesity. *Arch Int Med* 1976; 136:298.

DeSimone DP et al. Influence of body habitus and race on bone mineral density of the midradius, hip, and spine in aging women. *J Bone Miner Res* 1989; 4(6):827-830.

Ettinger B. Thyroid supplements: effect on bone mass. *West J Med* 1982; 136:473.

Felson DT et al. Thiazide diuretics and the risk of hip fracture: results from the Framingham study. *JAMA* 1991; 265(3):370-373.

Ferrini RL, Barrett-Connor E. Caffeine intake and endogenous sex steroid levels in postmenopausal women - The Rancho Bernardo Study. *Am J Epidem* 1996; 144:642-644.

Franklyn JA et al. Long-term thyroxine treatment and bone mineral density. *Lancet* 1992; 340:9-13.

Garnero P, Delmas PD. New developments in biochemical markers for osteoporosis. *Calcif Tissue Int* 1996; 59(suppl 1):52-59.

Gillespy M et al. Effect of long-term triphasic oral contraceptive use on glucose tolerance and insulin secretion. *Obstet Gynecol* 1991; 78(1):108-114

Gilsanz V et al. Vertebral bone density in children: effect of puberty. *Radiology* 1998; 166:847-850.

Gunson DE. Environmental zinc and cadmium pollution associated with general osteochrondrosis, osteoporosis and nephrocalcinosis in horses. *J Am Veterin Med Assn* 1982; 180:295.

Healey JH et al. Structural scoliosis in osteoporotic women. *Clin Ortho Rel Res 1985;* 195:216-223.

Heaney RP, Skillman TG. Calcium metabolism in normal human pregnancy. *J Clin Endocrinol Metab* 1971; 33:661.

Horowitz M et al. Treatment of postmenopausal hyperparathyroidism with norethindrone. *Arch Int Med* 1987; 147:681-685.

Howat PM et al. The effect of bulimia upon diet, body fat, bone density, and blood components. *J Am Dietetic Assn* 1989; 89:929-934.

Hreshchyshyn MM et al. Effects of natural menopause, hysterectomy, and oophorectomy on lumbar spine and femoral neck bone densities. *Obstet Gynecol* 1988; 72:631-638.

Johnston CC Jr, Longcope C. Premenopausal bone loss–a risk factor for osteoporosis. (editorial) *N Engl J Med* 1990; 323(18):1271-1272.

Johnston CC Jr et al. Risk assessment: theoretical considerations. *Am J Med* 1993; 95(suppl 5A): 2S-5S.

Kalkwarf H, Specker B. Bone mineral loss during lactation and recovery after weaning. *Obstet Gynecol* 1995; 86:26-32.

Kent GN et al. Human lactation: forearm trabecular bone loss, increased bone turnnover, and renal conservation of calcium and inorganic phosphate with recovery of bone mass following weaning. *J Bone Miner Res* 1990; 5(4):361-368.

Kiel DP et al. Smoking eliminates the protective effect of oral estrogens on the risk for hip fracture among women. *Ann Intern Med* 1992; 116:716-721.

Kleerekoper, M. Biochemical markers of bone remodeling. *Am J Med Sci* 1996; 312(6);270-277.

Klibanski A et al. Increase in bone mass after treatment of hyperprolactinemic amenorrhea. *N Engl J Med* 1986; 315:542-546.

Klibanski A et al. Decreased bone density in hyperprolactinemic women. *N Engl J Med* 1980; 303(26): 1511-1514, 1980.

Krall E, Dawson-Hughes B. Smoking and bone loss among postmenopausal women. *J Bone Miner Res* 1991; 6(4):331-337.

Kung AWC et al. Bone mineral density in premenopausal women receiving long-term physiological doses of levothyroxine. *JAMA* 1991; 265(20):2688-2691.

LaCroix AZ et al. Thiazide diuretic agents and the incidence of hip fracture. *N Engl J Med* 1990; 322: 286-290.

Lam SY et al. Gynaecological disorders and risk factors in premenopausal women predisposing to osteoporosis: a review. *Brit J Obstet Gynecol* 1988; 95:963-972.

Lane N et al. Rheumatoid arthritis and bone mineral density in elderly women. *J Bone Miner Res* 1995; 10(2):257-63.

Lindquist O, Bengtsson C. The effect of smoking on menopausal age. *Maturitas* 1979; 1:171.

Lindsay R. The influence of cigarette smoking on bone mass and bone loss. In *Osteoporosis: Recent Advances in Pathogenesis and Treatment*, HF DeLuca et al, eds. Baltimore, Maryland: University Park Press, 1981.

Lindsay R et al. Prevention of spinal osteoporosis in oophorectomised women. *Lancet* ii:1980; 1151-1154.

Lloyd T et al. Collegiate women athletes with irregular menses during adolescence have decreased bone density. *Obstet Gynecol* 1988; 72:639-642.

Lindsay R et al. Women athletes with menstrual irregularities have Increased musculoskeletal injuries. *Med and Sci Sports and Exercise* 1986; 18(4):374-379.

Martin P et al. Partially reversible osteopenia after surgery for primary hyperparathyroidism. *Arch Int Med* 1986; 146:689-691.

Miller P, McClung M. Prediction of fracture risk I: bone density. *Am J Med Sci* 1996;312(6):257-259.

Notelovitz M et al. The effect of low-dose oral contraceptives on lipids and lipoproteins in two at-risk populations: young female smokers and older premenopausal women. *Am J Obstet Gynecol* 1985; 152(8):995-1000.

Paul TL et al. Long-term L-thyroxine therapy is associated with decreased hip bone density in premenopausal women. *JAMA* 1988; 259(21): 3137-3141.

Prior JC et al. Spinal bone loss and ovulatory disturbances. *N Engl J Med* 1990; 323(18): 1221-1227.

Ray WA et al. Long-term use of thiazide diuretics and risk of hip fracture. *Lancet* i:687-690, 1989.

Rigotti NA et al. The clinical course of osteoporosis in anorexia nervosa: a longitudinal study of cortical bone mass. *JAMA* 1991; 265: 1133-1138.

Rigotti NA et al. Osteoporosis in women with anorexia nervosa. *N Engl J Med* 1984; 311(25): 1601-1606.

Rosen CJ et al. The predictive value of biochemical markers of bone turnover for bone mineral density in early postmenopausal women treated with hormone replacement or calcium supplementation. *J Clin Endocrinol Metab* 1997; 82:1904-1910.

Rosenthal DI et al. Age and bone mass in premenopausal women. *J Bone Miner Res* 1989; 4(4): 533-538.

Ross P. Prediction of fracture risk II: other risk factors. *Am J Med Sci* 1996; 312(6);260-269.

Schnitzler CM, Solomon L. Bone changes after alcohol abuse. *So African Med J* 1984; 66:730-734.

Seeman E et al. Reduced bone mass in daughters of women with osteoporosis. *N Engl J Med* 1989; 320:554-558.

Seeman E et al. Reduced femoral neck bone density in the daughters of women with hip fractures: The role of low peak bone density in the pathogenesis of osteoporosis. *J Bone Miner Res* 1994; 9(5):739-43.

Slemenda CW et al. Genetic determinants of bone mass in adult women: a reevaluation of the twin model and the potential importance of gene interaction on heritability estimates. *J Bone Miner Res* 1991; 6(6):561-567.

Smith DM et al. Genetic factors in determining bone mass. *J Clin Invest* 1973; 52:2800.

Smith R et al. Osteoporosis of pregnancy. *Lancet* 1985; i:1178-1180.

Soroko S et al. Family history of osteoporosis and bone mineral density at the axial skeleton: the rancho bernardo study. *J Bone Miner Res* 1994; 9(6):761-69.

Sowers M et al. Changes in bone density with lactation. *JAMA* 1993; 269(24):3130-3135.

Taitel H, Lippman J. Effects of oral contraceptives on bone mass. *The Female Patient* 1995; 20:38-55.

Tummons IS et al. Bone mineral density in women with endometriosis before and during ovarian suppression with gonadotropin-releasing hormone agonists or Danazol. *Fertil Steril* 1988; 49(5): 792-796.

Tuppurainen M et al. The effect of gynecological risk factors on lumbar and femoral bone mineral density in peri- and postmenopausal women. *Maturitas 1995;* 21:137-145.

Warren MP et al. Scoliosis and fractures in young ballet dancers: relation to delayed menarche and secondary amenorrhea. *N Engl J Med* 1986; 314:1348-1353.

Watson N et al. Bone loss after hysterectomy with ovarian conservation. *Obstet Gynecol* 1995; 86:72-77.

Weinstein RS, Bell NH. Diminished rates of bone formation in normal black adults. *N Engl J Med* 1988; 319:1698-1701.

Weinstock RS et al. Bone mineral density in women with type II diabetes mellitus. *J Bone Miner Res 1989;* 4(1):97-101.

Winter RB. Adolescent idiopathic scoliosis. *N Engl J Med* (editorial) 1986; 314(21):1379-1380.

CHAPTER 5

Antich PP et al. Measurement of mechanical properties of bone material in vitro by ultrasound reflection: methodology and comparison with ultrasound transmission. *J Bone Miner Res* 1991; 6(4):417-426.

Bauer D et al. Quantitative ultrasound and vertebral fracture in postmenopausal women. *J Bone Miner Res* 1995; 10(3):353-58.

Bevier WC et al. Relationship of body composition, muscle strength, and aerobic capacity to bone mineral density in older men and women. *J Bone Miner Res* 1989; 4(3):421-432.

Black DM et al. Comparison of methods for defining prevalent vertebral deformities: the study of osteoporotic fractures. *J Bone Miner Res* 1995; 10(6):890-902.

Black DM et al. Axial and appendicular bone density predict fractures in older women. *J Bone Miner Res* 1992; 7(6):633-638.

Black DM et al. Appendicular bone mineral and a woman's lifetime risk of hip fracture. *J Bone Miner Res* 1992; 7(6):639-646.

Burks D, Walsh B, Maricic M. Repeat bone densitometry affects patients decisions to continue osteoporosis medication. *Am Coll Rheumatol* 1995; 38:S357.

Carter DR et al. New approaches for interpreting projected bone densitometry data. *J Bone Miner Res* 1992; 7(2):137-145.

Clark AP, Schuttinga JA. Targeted estrogen/progestogen replacement therapy for osteoporosis: calculation of health care cost savings. *Osteo Int* 1992; 2:195-200.

Cook B et al. An osteoporosis patient education and screening program: results and implications. *Patient Ed Counseling* 1991; 17:135-145.

Cosman F et al. Radiographic absorptiometry: A simple method for determination of bone mass. *Osteo Int* 1991; 2:34-38.

Cummings SR et al. Appendicular bone density and age predict hip fracture in women. *JAMA* 1990; 263(5):665-668.

Cutler WB et al. Single photon absorptiometry imaging as a screening method for diminished dual photon density measures. *Maturitas* 1988; 10:143-155.

Delmas PD. Biochemical markers of bone turnover I: theoretical considerations and clinical use in osteoporosis. *Am J Med* 1993; 95(suppl 5A): 11S-16S.

Gertz B et al. Monitoring bone resorption in early postmenopausal women by an immunoassay for cross-linked collagen peptides in urine. *J Bone Miner Res* 1994; 9(2):135-142.

Gluer C et al. Prediction of hip fractures from pelvic radiographs: the study of osteoporotic fractures. *J Bone Miner Res* 1994; 9(5):671-77.

Heaney R et al. Ultrasound velocity through bone predicts incident vertebral deformity. *J Bone Miner Res* 1995; 10(3):341-45.

Heaney R et al. Osteoporotic bone fragility: detection by ultrasound transmission velocity. *JAMA* 1989; 261(20):2986-2990.

Johnston CC Jr et al. Clinical use of bone densitometry. *N Engl J Med* 1991; 324(16):1105-1109.

Johnston CC Jr et al. Clinical indications for bone mass measurements: a report from the scientific advisory board of the National Osteoporosis Foundation. *J Bone Miner Res* 1989; 4(suppl 2):1-28.

Kanis J et al. Perspective the diagnosis of osteoporosis. *J Bone Miner Res* 1994; 9(8):1137-41.

Kanis JA. Osteoporosis and osteopenia. *J Bone Miner Res* (editorial) 1990; 5(3):209-211.

Langton CM et al. The measurement of broadband ultrasonic attenuation in cancellous bone. *Engineering in Med* 1984; 13(2):89-91.

Leboff MS et al. Dual-energy x-ray absorptiometry of the forearm: reproducibility and correlation with sIngle-photon absorptiometry. *J Bone Miner Res* 1992; 7(7):841-846.

Lydick E et al. Development and validation of a simple questionnaire to facilitate identification of women with low bone density. *J Bone Miner Res* 1996; 11:(suppl 1):S368.

Melton LJ III et al. Screening for osteoporosis. *Ann Intern Med* 1990; 112:516-528.

National Osteoporosis Foundation Working Group on Vertebral Fractures: report assessing vertebral fractures. *J Bone Miner Res* 1995; 10(4):518-23, 1995.

Orwoll ES et al. Longitudinal precision of dual-energy x-ray absorptiometry in a multicenter study. *J Bone Miner Res* 1991; 6(2):191-197.

Overgaard K, Christiansen C. A new biochemical marker of bone resorption for follow-up on treatment with nasal salmon calcitonin. *Calcif Tissue Int* 1996; 59:12 16.

Pocock NA et al. Muscle strength, physical fitness, and weight but not age predict femoral neck bone mass. *J Bone Miner Res* 1989; 4(3):441-448.

Pocock NA et al. Physical fitness is a major determinant of femoral neck and lumbar spine mineral density. *J Clin Inv* 1986; 78:618-621.

Ravn P et al. High bone turnover is associated with low bone mass in both pre- and postmenopausal women. *Bone* 1996; 19:291-298.

Reid DM et al. Perimenopausal osteoporosis screening: the effectiveness of direct disclosure of results. *Bone* 1997; 20:6S.

Riis BJ. Biochemical markers of bone turnover II: diagnosis, prophylaxis, and treatment of osteoporosis. *Am J Med* 1993; 95(suppl 5A): 17S-21S.

Riis BJ et al. Low bone mass and fast rate of bone loss at menopause: equal risk factors for future fracture: a 15-year follow-up study. *Bone* 1996; 19:9-12.

Ross PD et al. Detection of prefracture spinal osteoporosis using bone mineral absorptiometry. *J Bone Miner Res* 1988; 3(1):1-11.

Schott A et al. Ultrasound discriminates patients with hip fracture equally well as dual energy x-ray absorptiometry and independently of bone mineral density. *J Bone Miner Res* 1995; 10(2): 243-49.

Snow-Harter C et al. Muscle strength as a predictor of bone mineral density in young women. *J Bone Miner Res* 1990; 5(6):589-595.

Sowers MR et al. Radial bone mineral density in pre- and perimenopausal women: a prospective study of rates and risk factors for loss. *J Bone Miner Res* 1992; 7(6):647-657.

Stegman M et al. Comparison of speed of sound ultrasound with single photon absorptiometry for determining fracture odds ratios. *J Bone Miner Res* 1995; 10(3):346-52.

Steiger P et al. Age-related decrements in bone mineral density in women over 65. *J Bone Miner Res* 1992; 7(6):625-632.

Tesar R, Notelovitz M, Harris W. Single photon absorptiometry—a valid method for detecting osteopenia, abstract no. 145. *Maturitas* 1984; 6:107.

Tosteson ANA et al. Cost effectiveness of screening perimenopausal white women for osteoporosis: bone densitometry and hormone replacement therapy. *Ann Intern Med* 1990; 113:594-603.

Uebelhart F et al. Lateral dual-photon sbsorptiometry: a new technique to measure the bone mineral density at the lumbar spine. *J Bone Miner Res* 1990; 5(5):525-531.

vanHemert AM et al. Prediction of osteoporotic fractures in the general population by a fracture risk score. *Am J Epidem* 1990; 132(1): 123-134.

Wasnich RD et al. Prediction of postmenopausal fracture risk with use of bone mineral measurements. *Am J Obstet Gynecol* 1985; 153: 745-751.

Wasnich RD. Bone mass measurement: prediction of risk. *Am J Med* 1993; 95(suppl 5A):6S-10S.

CHAPTER 6

Anderson JJB, Rondano PA. Peak bone mass development of females: can young adult women improve their peak bone mass? *J Am Coll Nutr* 1996; 15:570-574.

Avioli LV. Calcium and osteoporosis. *Annual Rev Nutrit* 1984; 4:471-491.

Chapuy MC et al. Vitamin D3 and calcium to prevent hip fractures in elderly women. *N Engl J Med* 1992; 327(23):1637-1642.

Curhan GC et al. A prospective study of dietary calcium and other nutrients and the risk of symptomatic kidney stones. *N Engl J Med* 1993; 328(12):833-838.

Cumming RG, Nevitt MC. Calcium for prevention of osteoporotic fractures in postmenopausal women. *J Bone Miner Res* 1997; 12:1321.

Dawson-Hughes B et al. A controlled trial of the effect of calcium supplementation on bone density in postmenopausal women. *N Engl J Med* 1990; 323(13):878-883.

Dawson-Hughes B et al. Effect of calcium and vitamin D supplementation on bone density in men and women 65 years of age or older. *N Engl J Med* 1997; 337:670-6.

Dawson-Hughes B et al. Sodium excretion influences calcium homeostasis in elderly men and women. *J Nutr* 1996; 126:2107-2112.

Favus MJ. Intestinal calcium absorption: have we absorbed enough from research to have a test for the patient? *J Bone Miner Res* (editorial) 1989; 4(4):461-462.

Finkenstedt G et al. Lactose absorption, milk consumption, and fasting blood glucose concentrations in women with idiopathic osteoporosis. *Br Med J* 1986; 292:161-162.

Food and Nutrition Board, Institute of Medicine: *Dietary reference intakes for calcium, phosphorus, magnesium, vitamin D and fluoride.* Washington, D.C.: National Academy Press, 1997

Garland C et al. Dietary vitamin D and calcium and risk of colorectal cancer: a 19-year prospective study in men. *Lancet* 1985; i:307-309.

Hansen C et al. Intestinal calcium absorption from different calcium preparations: influence of anion and solubility. *Osteoporosis Int* 1996; 6: 386-393.

Heaney RP. Bone mass, nutrition, and other lifestyle factors. *Am J Med* 95(suppl 5A):29S-33S.

Heaney RP. Thinking straight about calcium. *N Engl J Med* (editorial) 1993; 328(7):503-504.

Heaney RP. Pathophysiology of osteoporosis. *Am J Med Sci* 1996; 312:251-256.

Heaney RP et al. Calcium absorption in women: relationships to calcium intake, estrogen status, and age. *J Bone Miner Res* 1989; 4(4):469-475.

Heaney RP et al. Calcium nutrition and bone health in the elderly. *Am J Clin Nutrition* 1982; 36:986-1013.

Heaney RP, Weaver CM. Calcium absorption from kale. *Am J Clin Nutrition* 1990; 51:656-657.

Hill PB et al. Gonadotrophin release and meat consumption in vegetarian women. *Am J Clin Nutrition* 1986; 43:37-41.

Holbrook TL et al. Dietary calcium and risk of hip fracture: 14-year prospective population study. *Lancet* ii:1988; 1046-1049.

Itoh, Suyama. Sodium and calcium. *Am J Clin Nutrition* 1996 (63):735-40.

Johnston CC Jr et al. Calcium supplementation and increases in bone mineral density in children. *N Engl J Med* 1992; 327:82-87.

Kanders B et al. Interaction of calcium nutrition and physical activity on bone mass in young women. *J Bone Miner Res* 1988; 3(2):145-149.

Lactase deficiency in osteoporosis. Editorial. *Lancet* 1979; i:86.

Lemann J Jr. Composition of the diet and calcium kidney stones. *N Engl J Med* (editorial) 1993; 328(12):880-881.

Lips, P. Vitamin D deficiency and osteoporosis: the role of vitamin D deficiency and treatment with vitamin D and analogues in the prevention of osteoporosis-related fractures. *Eur J Clin Invest* 1996; 26:436-442.

Lloyd T et al. The effect of calcium supplementation and Tanner stage on bone density, content and area in teenage women. *Osteoporosis Int.* 1996; 6:276-283.

Marsh AG et al. Vegetarian lifestyle and bone mineral density. *Am J Clin Nutrition* 1988; 48:837-41.

Matkovic V. Calcium intake and peak bone mass. *N Engl J Med* (editorial) 1992; 327(2):119-120.

Matkovic V et al. Factors that influence peak bone mass formation: a study of calcium balance and the inheritance of bone mass in adolescent females. *Am J Clin Nutr* 1990; 52:878-888.

Newcomer AD et al. Lactase deficiency: prevalence in osteoporosis. *Ann Intern Med* 1978; 89:218-220.

Notelovitz M. Estrogen therapy and osteoporosis: principles and practice. *Am J Med Sci* 1997; 313:2-12.

Parfitt AM. Dietary risk factors for age-related bone loss and fractures. *Lancet* ii:1983; 1181-1184.

Prince RL. et al. The pathogenesis of age-related osteoporotic fracture: Effects of dietary calcium deprivation. *J Clin Endocrinol Metab* 1997; 82:260-264.

Punnonen R et al. Serum 25-OHD, vitamin A and vitamin E concentrations in healthy Finnish and Floridian women. *Int J Vit Nutrition Res* 1988; 58:37-39.

Recker RR et al. Correcting calcium nutritional deficiency prevents spine fractures in elderly women. *J Bone Miner Res* 1996; 11:1961-1966.

Reid I. Therapy of osteoporosis: calcium, vitamin D, and exercise. *Am J Med Sci* 1996; 312(6): 278-286.

Reid IR et al. Effect of calcium supplementation on bone loss in postmenopausal women. *N Engl J Med* 1993; 328(7):460-464.

Silverman SL. Calcitonin. *Am J Med Sci* 1997; 313:13-16.

Spencer H et al. Calcium requirements in humans: report of original data and a review. *Clin Ortho Rel Res* 1984; 184:270-280.

Tesar R et al. Axial and peripheral bone density and nutrient intakes of postmenopausal women and omnivorous women. *Am J Clin Nutr* 1992; 56:699-704.

Utiger, RD. The need for more vitamin D. *N Engl J Med* 1998; 338:828-829.

van der Wielen R et al. Serum vitamin D concentrations among elderly people in Europe. *Lancet* 1995; 346:207-210.

CHAPTER 7

Bell NH et al. The effects of muscle-building exercise on vitamin D and mineral metabolism. *J Bone Miner Res* 1988; 3(4):369-373.

Blimkie CJR et al. Effects of resistance training on bone mineral content and density in adolescent females. *Can J Physiol Pharmacol* 1996; 74:1025-1033.

Boot AM et al. Bone mineral density in children and adolescents: relation to puberty, calcium intake, and physical activity. *J Clin Endocrin Metab* 1997; 82:57-62.

Bush TL et al. Effects of hormone therapy on bone mineral density: results from the postmenopausal estrogen/ progestin interventions (PEPI) trial. *JAMA* 1996; 276:1389-1396.

Cooper C et al. Childhood growth, physical activity, and peak bone mass in women. *J Bone Miner Res* 1995; 10(6):940-47.

Dalsky GP et al. Weight-bearing exercise training and lumbar bone mineral content in post-menopausal women. *Ann Intern Med* 1988; 108:824-828, 1988.

Davee AM et al. Exercise patterns and trabecular bone density in college women. *J Bone Miner Res* 1990; 5(3):245-250.

Drinkwater BL et al. Bone mineral density after resumption of menses in amenorrheic athletes. *JAMA* 1986; 256(3):380-382.

Drinkwater BL et al. Menstrual history as a determinant of current bone density in young athletes. *JAMA* 1990; 263(4):545-548.

Etherington J et al. The effect of weight-bearing exercise on bone mineral density: a study of female ex-elite athletes and the general population. *J Bone Miner Res* 1996; 11:1333-1338.

Friedlander A et al. A two-year program of aerobics and weight training enhances bone mineral density of young women. *J Bone Miner Res* 1995; 10(4):574-85.

Gleeson PB et al. Effects of weight lifting on bone mineral density in premenopausal women. *J Bone Miner Res* 1990; 5(2):153-158.

Heinrich CH et al. Bone mineral content of cyclically menstrurating female resistance and endurance trained athletes. *Med Sci Sports Exer* 1990; 22(5):558-563.

Huddleston AL et al. Bone mass in lifetime tennis athletes. *JAMA* 244(10):1107-1109, 1980.

Johnston CCJr, Longcope C. Premenopausal bone loss–a risk factor for osteoporosis. Editorial. *N Engl J Med* 1990; 323(18):1271-1272.

Kanders B et al. Interaction of calcium nutrition and physical activity on bone mass in young women. *J Bone Miner Res* 1988; 3(2):145-149.

Kelly JB, Hatfield SL. Menstrual irregularities and bone loss in female athletes. *The Female Patient* 1989; 14:35-39.

Kohrt W et al. Additive effects of weight-bearing exercise and estrogen on bone mineral density in older women. *J Bone Miner Res* 1995; 10(9): 1303-11.

Lindberg JS et al. Exercise-induced amenorrhea and bone density. *Ann Intern Med 1984; 101(5):* 647-648.

Linnell SL et al. Bone mineral content and menstrual regularity in female runners. *Med Sci Sports Exer 1984;* 16(4):343-348.

Lohman T et al. Effects of resistance training on regional and total bone mineral density in premenopausal women: a randomized prospective study. *J Bone Miner Res* 1995; 10(7): 1015-24.

Lord SR et al. The effects of a community exercise program on fracture risk factors in older women. *Osteoporosis Int* 1996; 6:361-367.

Martin D, Notelovitz M. Effects of aerobic training on bone mineral density of postmenopausal women. *J Bone Miner Res* 1993; 8(8):931-936.

Notelovitz M et al. Cardiorespiratory fitness evaluation in climacteric women: comparison of two methods. *Am J Obstet Gynecol* 1986; 54(5): 1009-1013.

Notelovitz M et al. Estrogen therapy and variable-resistance weight training increase bone mineral in surgically menopausal women. *J Bone Miner Res* 1991; 6(6):583-590.

Orwoll ES et al. The relationship of swimming exercise to bone mass in men and women. *Arch Int Med* 1989; 149:2197-2200.

Osteoporosis and activity. Editorial. *Lancet* 1983; i:1365-1366.

Prince R et al. The effects of calcium supplementation (milk powder or tablets) and exercise on bone density in postmenopausal women. *J Bone Miner Res 1995;* 10(7):1068-75.

Prince R et al. Prevention of postmenopausal osteoporosis: a comparative study of exercise, calcium supplementation, and hormone-replacement therapy. *N Engl J Med* 1991; 325(17): 1189-1195.

Province MA et al. The effects of exercise on falls in elderly patients. *JAMA* 1995; 273:1341-1347.

Pruitt LA et al. Effects of a one-year high-intensity versus low-intensity resistance training program on bone mineral density in older women. *J Bone Miner Res* 1995; 10(11):1788-1795.

Recker RR et al. Bone gain in young adult women. *JAMA* 1992; 268(17):2403-2408.

Reid I. Therapy of osteoporosis: calcium, vitamin D, and exercise. *Am J Med Sci* 1996; 312(6): 278-286.

Ruiz J et al. Influence of spontaneous calcium intake and physical exercise on the vertebral and femoral bone mineral density of children and adolescents. *J Bone Miner Res* 1995; 10(5):675-82.

Shangold M et al. Evaluation and management of menstrual dysfunction in athletes. *JAMA* 1990; 263(12):1665-1669.

Snow-Harter C et al. Effects of resistance and endurance exercise on bone mineral status of young women: a randomized exercise intervention trial. *J Bone Miner Res* 1992; 7(7):761-769.

Taaffe D et al. Differential effects of swimming versus weight-bearing activity on bone mineral status of eumenorrheic athletes. *J Bone Miner Res* 1995; 10(4):586-93.

Taaffe D et al. High-impact exercise promotes bone gain in well-trained female athletes. *J Bone Miner Res* 1997; 12:255-260.

CHAPTER 8

Aloia JF et al. Treatment of osteoporosis with calcitonin, with and without growth hormone. *Metabolism* 1985; 34(2):124-129.

Avioli LV. Calcitonin therapy for bone disease and hypercalcemia. *Arch Int Med* 1982; 142:2076-2079.

Brandi ML. New treatment strategies: ipriflavone, strontium, vitamin D metabolites and analogs. *Am J Med* 1993; 95(suppl 5A):69S-74S.

Burks D et al. Repeat bone densitometry affects patients decisions to continue osteoporosis medication. *Am Coll Rheumatol* 1995; 38:S357.

Chesnut CH et al. Alendronate treatment of the postmenopausal osteoporotic woman: effect of multiple dosages on bone mass and bone remodeling. *Am J Med* 1995; 99:144-152.

Compston JE. The therapeutic use of bisphosphonates. *Br Med J* 1994; 309:711-15.

Danielson C et al. Hip fractures and fluoridation in Utah's elderly population. *JAMA* 1992; 268(6): 746-748.

Davis S et al. Testosterone enhances estradiol's effects on postmenopausal bone density and sexuality. *Maturitas* 1995; 21:227-36.

Fatourechi V, Heath H. Salmon calcitonin in the treatment of postmenopausal osteoporosis. Editorial. *Ann Intl Med* 1987; 107(6):923-925.

Hammar MD et al. Effects of hormone replacement therapy on the postural balance among postmenopausal women. *Obstet Gynecol* 1996; 88: 955-960.

Hosking D. Prevention of bone loss with alendronate in postmenopausal women under 60 years of age. *N Engl J Med* 1998; 338:485-92.

Hurley DL. Axial and appendicular bone mineral density in patients with long-term deficiency or excess of calcitonin. *N Engl J Med* 1987; 317(9): 537-541.

Jones G et al. Thiazide diuretics and fractures: can meta-analysis help? *J Bone Miner Res* 1995; 10(1): 106-11.

Kanis JA. Treatment of symptomatic osteoporosis with fluoride. *Am J Med* 1993; 95(suppl 5A): 53S-61S.

Lieberman UA et al. Effect of oral alendronate on bone mineral density and the incidence of fractures in postmenopausal osteoporosis. *N Engl J Med* 1995; 333:1437-43.

Lindsay R. Fluoride and bone–quantity versus quality. *N Engl J Med* 1990; 322(12):845-846.

Lueg MC. Postmenopausal osteoporosis: treatment with low-dose sodium fluoride and estrogen. *Southern Med J* 1988; 81(5):597-600.

MacIntyre I et al. Calcitonin for prevention of postmenopausal bone loss. *Lancet* 1988; i:900-901.

Mamelle N et al. Risk-benefit ratio of sodium fluoride treatment in primary vertebral osteoporosis. *Lancet* ii:1988; 361-365.

New treatments for osteoporosis. Editorial. *Lancet* 1990; 355:1065-1066.

Notelovitz, M. Estrogen therapy and osteoporosis: principles and practice. *Am J Med Sci* 1997; 313(1):2-12.

Overgaard K et al. Discontinuous calcitonin treatment of established osteoporosis – effects of withdrawal treatment. *Am J Med* 1990; 89:1-6.

Overgaard K et al. Patient responsiveness to calcitonin salmon nasal spray. *The Female Patient* Oct 1995; supp 1-4.

Pak et al. Intermittent fluoride plus calcium strengthens bone. *J Musculoskeletal Med* Dec. 1994:63.

Papapoulos SE. The role of bisphosphonates in the prevention and treatment of osteoporosis. *Am J Med* 1993; 95(suppl 5A):48S-51S.

Reginster JY et al. One-year controlled randomised trial of prevention of early postmenopausal bone loss by intranasal calcitonin. *Lancet* 1987; ii:1481-1483.

Reginster JY et al. Prevention of postmenopausal bone loss by Tiludronate. *Lancet* 1989; ii:1469-1471.

Riggs BL. A new option for treating osteoporosis. Editorial. *N Engl J Med* 1990; 323(2):124-125.

Riggs BL et al. Effect of fluoride treatment on the fracture rate in postmenopausal women with osteoporosis. *N Engl J Med* 1990; 322:802-809.

Riggs BL et al. Effect of the fluoride/calcium regimen on vertebral fracture occurrence in post-menopausal osteoporosis. *N Engl J Med* 1982; 306:446-450.

Riggs BL, Melton LJ. The prevention and treatment of osteoporosis. *N Engl J Med* 327(9): 1992; 620-627.

Reid DM et al. Perimenopausal osteoporosis screening: the effectiveness of direct disclosure of results. *Bone* 1997; 20:6S.

Rodan GA, Balena R. Bisphosphonates in the treatment of metabolic bone diseases. *Annals Med* 1993; 25:373-8.

Silverman SS et al. Effect of bone density information on decisions about hormone replacement therapy: a randomized trial. *Obstet Gynecol* 1997; 89:321-325.

Storm T et al. Effect of intermittent cyclical etidronate therapy on bone mass and fracture rate in women with postmenopausal osteoporosis. *N Engl J Med* 1990; 322:1265-1271.

Wallach S. Calcitonin treatment in osteoporosis. *The Female Patient* 1992; 17:35-50.

Watts NB et al. Intermittent cyclical etidronate treatment of postmenopausal osteoporosis. *N Engl J Med* 1990; 323(2):73-79.

Zhang Y et al. Bone mass and the risk of breast cancer among postmenopausal women. *N Engl J Med* 1997; 336:611-617.

CHAPTER 9

Abulla HI et al. Prevention of bone mineral loss in postmenopausal women by norethisterone. *Obstet Gynecol* 1985; 66:789-792.

Aitken, JJ et al. Oestrogen replacement therapy for prevention of osteoporosis after oophorectomy. *Br Med J* 1973; 3:515.

Burkman RT. Non-contraceptive effects of hormonal contraceptives: bone mass, sexually transmitted disease and pelvic inflammatory disease, cardiovascular disease, menstrual function and future fertility. *Am J Obstet Gynecol* 1994; 170:1569-1575.

Chen TL et al. Glucocorticoid receptors and inhibition of bone cell growth in primary culture. *Endocrinology* 1977; 100:619-628.

Christiansen C et al. Prevention of early post-menopausal bone loss: controlled 2-year study in 315 normal females. *Eur J Clin Invest* 1980; 10:273.

Christiansen C et al. Bone mass in postmenopausal women after withdrawal of oestrogen/gestagen replacement therapy. *Lancet* 1981; 1:459-461.

Christiansen C, Lindsay R. Estrogens, bone loss and preservation. *Osteo Int* 1990; 1:7-13.

Christiansen C, Riis BJ. 17B estradiol and continuous norethisterone: a unique treatment for established osteoporosis in elderly women. *J Clin Endocrinol Metab* 1990; 71:836-841.

Christiansen MS et al. Dose-response evaluation of cyclic estrogen-gestagen in post-menopausal women: placebo-controlled trial of its gynecologic and metabolic actions. *Am J Obstet Gynecol* 1982; 144:873-879, 1982.

Cumming, Robert G, Mitchell, Paul. Hormone replacement therapy, reproductive factors, and cataract: The blue mountain eye study. *AmJEpidemiol* 1997; 145(3):242-249.

DeCree C et al. Suitability of cyproterone acetate in the treatment of osteoporosis associated with athletic amenorrhea. *Int J Sports Med* 1988; 9:187-192.

del Castillo et al. Effects of estrogen use on lens transmittance in postmenopausal women. *Ophthalmology* 1997; 104:970-973.

Dupont WD, Page DL. Menopausal estrogen replacement therapy and breast cancer. *Arch Intern Med* 1991; 151:67-72.

Ericksen EF et al. Evidence of estrogen receptors in normal human osteoblast-like cells. *Science* 1988; 241:84-86.

Ettinger B et al. Long-term estrogen replacement therapy prevents bone loss and fractures. *Ann Intern Med* 1985; 102:319-324.

Ettinger B et al. Low-dosage estrogen combined with calcium prevents postmenopausal bone loss: results of a three-year study. In Cohn DV et al, eds. *Calcium Regulation and Bone Metabolism: Basic and Clinical Aspects.* Amsterdam: Elsevier, 1987; 918-922.

Ettinger B et al. Low-dosage micronized 17B-estrodiol prevents bone loss in post-menopausal women. *Am J Obstet Gynecol* 1992; 166:479-488.

Felson DT et al. The effect of postmenopausal estrogen on bone density in elderly women. *N Engl J Med* 1993; 329:1141-1146.

Field CS et al. Preventive effects of transdermal 17B-estradiol on osteoporotic changes after surgical menopause: a two-year placebo-controlled trial. *Am J Obstet Gynecol* 1993; 168: 114-121.

Gallagher JC et al. Effect of progestin therapy on cortical and trabecular bone: comparison with estrogen. *Am J Med* 1991; 90:171-178.

Gambacciani M et al. Longitudinal evaluation of perimenopausal vertebral bone loss: effects of a low-dose oral contraceptive preparation on bone mineral density and metabolism. *Obstet Gynecol* 1994; 83:392-396.

Gambrell RD et al. Estrogen therapy and breast cancer in postmenopausal women. *J Am Geriatrics Soc* 1980; 28:251.

Gambrell RD et al. Reduced incidence of endometrial cancer among postmenopausal women treated with progestogens. *J Am Geriatrics Soc* 1979; 27:389.

Genant HK et al. Effect of estrone sulphate on postmenopausal bone loss. *Obstet Gynecol* 1990; 76:579-584.

Genant HK et al. Low-dose esterified estrogen therapy: effects on bone, plasma estradiol concentrations, endometrium, and lipid levels. *Arch Intern Med* 1997; 157:2609-2615.

Geola FL et al. Biological effects of various doses of conjugated equine estrogens in postmenopausal women. *J Clin Endocrinol Metab* 1980; 51:620.

Holland EFN et al. Histomorphometric changes in

the skeleton of postmenopausal women with low bone mineral density treated with percutaneous estradiol implants. *Obstet Gynecol* 1994; 83:387-391.

Horsman A et al. The effect of estrogen dose on postmenopausal bone loss. *N Engl J Med* 1983; 309:1405-1407.

Horsman A et al. Prospective trial of oestrogen and calcium in postmenopausal women. *Br Med J* 1977; 2:789.

Hulka BS et al. Breast cancer and estrogen replacement therapy. *Am J Obstet Gynecol* 1982; 143: 638.

Hutchinson TA et al. Post-menopausal oestrogens protect against fractures of hip and distal radius. *Lancet* 1979; 2:705.

Klein, Barbara EK et al. Is there evidence of an estrogen effect on age-related lens opacities? The beaver dam eye study. *Arch Ophthal* 1994; 112:85-91

Lindsay R et al. Bone response to termination of oestrogen treatment. *Lancet* 1:1325, 1978.

Lindsay R et al. Comparative effects of oestrogen and a progestogen on bone mass in postmenopausal women. *Clin Sci Molec Med* 1978; 54:193.

Lindsay R et al. Estrogen treatment of patients with established postmenopausal osteoporosis. *Obstet Gynecol* 1990; 76:290-295.

Lindsay R et al. Long-term prevention of postmenopausal osteoporosis by oestrogen. *Lancet* 1976; 1:1038.

Lindsay R et al. The minimum effective dose of estrogen for prevention of postmenopausal bone loss. *Obstet Gynecol* 1984; 63:759-763.

Lindsay R et al. Prevention of spinal osteoporosis in oophorectomized women. *Lancet* 1980; 2:1151.

Lufkin EG, et al. Treatment of postmenopausal osteoporosis with transdermal estrogen. *Ann Intern Med* 1992; 117:1-9.

Marshall RW et al. The effect of ethinyloestradiol on calcium and bone metabolism in peri-and postmenopausal women. *Horm Metab Res.* 1984; 16:97-99.

Mazess RB et al. Monitoring skeletal response to estrogen. *Am J Obstet Gynecol* 1989; 1(4):843-848.

Meema HE, Meema S. Prevention of postmenopausal osteoporosis by hormone treatment of the menopause. *Can Med Assn J* 1968; 99:248.

Meema S et al. Preventive effect of estrogen on postmenopausal bone loss. *Arch Int Med* 1975; 135:1436.

Moore M et al. Long-term estrogen replacement therapy in postmenopausal women sustains vertebral bone mineral density. *J Bone Miner Res* 1990; 5:659-663.

Munk-Jensen N et al. Reversal of postmenopausal vertebral bone loss by oestrogen and progestogen: a double blind, placebo controlled study. *Br Med J* 1988; 296:1150-1152.

Nachtigall LE et al. Estrogen replacement therapy. A 10-year prospective study in the relationship to osteoporosis. *Obstet Gynecol* 1979; 53: 277.

Nordin BEC et al. Treatment of spinal osteoporosis in postmenopausal women. *Br Med J* 1980; 280:251.

Notelovitz M. Osteoporosis screening, prevention and management. *Fertil Steril* 1993; 59:707-725.

Notelovitz M. Estrogen replacement therapy: indications, contraindications, and agent selection. *Am J Obstet Gynecol* 1989; 161(6):8-17.

Notelovitz M et al. Metabolic and hormonal effects of 25-mg and 50-mg 17 beta-estradiol implants in surgically menopausal women. *Obstet Gynecol* 1987; 70(5):749-754.

Notelovitz M et al. Effect of cyclic estrone sulfate treatment on lipid profiles of postmenopausal women with elevated cholesterol levels. *Obstet Gynecol* 1990; 76(1):65-70.

Prior JC. Progesterone as a bone-trophic hormone. *Endocr Rev* 1990; 11:386-398.

Recker RR et al. Effect of estrogens and calcium carbonate on bone loss in postmenopausal women. *Ann Intern Med* 1977; 87:649.

Riggs BL, Melton LJ. The prevention and treatment of osteoporosis. *N Engl J Med* 1992; 80:1261-1269.

Salmi T. Risk factors in endometrial carcinoma. *Acta Obstetricia et Gynecologica Scandinavia.* 1979; supplement 86.

Sellers TA et al. The role of hormone replacement therapy in the risk for breast cancer and total mortality in women with a family history of breast cancer. *Ann Intern Med* 1997 Dec 1; 127; 973-80.

Slemenda C et al. Sex steroids and bone mass: a study of changes about the time of menopause. *J Clin Invest* 1987; 80:1261-1269.

Stevenson JC et al. Effects of transdermal versus oral hormone replacement therapy on bone density in spine and proximal femur in postmenopausal women. *Lancet* 1990; 335: 265-269.

Studd J et al. The relationship between plasma estradiol and the increase in the bone density in postmenopausal women after treatment with subcutaneous hormone implants. *Am J Obstet Gynecol* 1990; 163:1474-1479.

Weiss NS et al. Decreased risk of fractures of the hip and lower forearm with postmenopausal use of estrogen *N Engl J Med* 1980; 303(21): 1195-1198.

Williams SR et al. A study of combined continuous ethinyl estradiol and norethindrone acetate for postmenopausal hormone replacement. *Am J Obstet Gynecol* 1990; 162:438-446.

CHAPTER 10

Battmann A et al. Serum fluoride and serum osteocalcin levels in response to a novel sustained-release monofluorophosphate preparation: comparison with plain monofluorophosphate. *Osteoporosis Int* 1997; 7:48-51.

Bjarnason NH et al. Tibolone: prevention of bone loss in late postmenopausal women. *J Clin Endocrinol Metab* 1996; 81:2419-2422.

Black DM et al. Randomized trial of effect of alendronate on risk of fracture in women with existing vertebral fractures. *Lancet* 1996; 348:1535-1541.

Cardona JM, Pastor E. Calcitonin versus etidronate for the treatment of postmenopausal osteoporosis: a meta-analysis of published clinical trials. *Osteoporosis Int* 1997; 7:165-174.

Delmas PD. Bisphosphonates in the treatment of bone diseases. *N Eng J Med* 1996; 335:1836-1837.

Delmas P et al. Effects of raloxifene on bone mineral density, serum cholesterol concentrations, and uterine endometrium in postmenopausal women. *New Eng J Med* 1997; 337:1641-1647.

Fleish H. Bisphosphonates: mechanisms of action and clinical use in osteoporosis an update. *Horm Metab Res* 1997; 29:145-150.

Gillin JC. The long and short of sleeping pills. Editorial. *N Engl J Med* 1991; 324(24):1735-1737.

Greenblatt DJ et al. Sensitivity to triazolam in the elderly. *N Engl J Med* 1991; 324(24):1691-1698.

Grisso JA et al. Risk ractors for falls as a cause of hip fracture in women. *N Engl J Med* 1991; 324(19):1326-1331.

Karpf DB et al. Prevention of nonvertebral fractures by alendronate. *JAMA* 1997; 277:1159-1164.

Lauritzen JB et al. Effect of external hip protectors on hip fractures. *Lancet* 1993; 341:11-13.

Liberman UA et al. Effect of oral alendronate on bone mineral density and the incidence of fractures in postmenopausal osteoporosis. *N Engl J Med* 1995; 333:1437-1443.

Licata, A. Bisphosphonate therapy. *Am J Med Sci* 1997; 313(1):17-22.

Lipsitz LA. Orthostatic hypotension in the elderly. *N Engl J Med* 1989; 321(14):952-957.

Lufkin EG et al. Raloxifene treatment of postmenopausal osteoporosis. *J Bone Miner Res* 1997; 12(suppl 1):S150.

Meunier PJ. Prevention of hip fractures. *Am J Med* 95(suppl 5A):75S-78S.

Nevitt MC et al. Risk factors for recurrent nonsyncopal falls. *JAMA* 1989; 261(18):2663-2668.

Pak C et al. Sustained-release sodium fluoride in the management of established postmenopausal osteoporosis. *Am J Med Sci* 1997; 313(1):23-32.

Pak C et al. Comparison of nonrandomized triails with slow-release sodium fluoride with a randomized placebo-controlled trial in post-menopausal osteoporosis. *J Bone Miner Res* 1996; 11:160-168.

Province M et al. The effects of exercise on falls in elderly patients. *JAMA* 1995; 273(17):1341-53.

Ravn P et al. The effect on bone mass and bone markers of different doses of ibandronate: a new bisphosphonate for prevention and treatment of postmenopausal osteoporosis: a 1-year, randomized, double-blind, placebo-controlled dose-finding study. *Bone* 1996;19:527-533.

Ray W A et al. Benzodiazepines of long and short elimination half-life and the risk of hip fracture. *JAMA* 1989; 262(23):3303-3307.

Ray W A et al. Psychotropic drug use and the risk of hip fracture. *N Engl J Med* 1987; 316(7): 363-369.

Reginster J. Miscellaneous and experimental agents. *Am J Med Sci* 1997; 313(1):33-40.

Rodan GA. Bone mass homeostasis and bisphosphonate action. *Bone* 1997; 20:1-4.

Sebaldt RJ et al. Comparison of etidronate and estrogen on lumbar spinal bone mineral density changes and vertebral fracture rate. *Bone* 1997; 20:102S.

Selby P. Alendronate treatment for osteoporosis: a review of the clinical evidence. *Osteoporosis Int* 1996; 6:419-426.

Silverman, S. Calcitonin. *Am J Med Sci* 1997; 313(1):13-16.

Sinaki M, Mikkelsen BA. Postmenopausal spinal osteoporosis: flexion vs extension exercises. *Arch Phys Med and Rehab* 1984; 65:277-280.

Stock JL et al. Calcitonin-salmon nasal spray reduces the incidence of new vertebral fractures in postmenopausal women: 3-year interim results of the Proof study. *J Bone Miner Res* 1997; 12(suppl 1):S149.

Storm T et al. Five years of clinical experience with intermittent cyclical etidronate for post-menopausal osteoporosis. *J Rheumatol* 1996; 23:1560-1564.

Tinetti ME et al. A multifactorial intervention to reduce the risk of falling among elderly people living in the community. *N Engl J Med* Sept. 1994; 331(13):821-28.

Tinetti ME et al. Risk factors for falls among elderly persons living in the community. *N Engl J Med* 1988; 319(26):1701-1707.

Tinetti ME et al. Predictors and prognosis of inability to get up after falls among elderly persons. *JAMA* 1993; 269(1):65-70.

Watts NB et al. Seven years of cyclical etidronate: continued improvement in spine BMD and progressive decline in vertebral fracture incidence. *Bone* 1995; 17:597-618.

CHAPTER 11

Bendavid EJ et al. Factors associated with bone mineral density in middle- aged men. *J Bone Miner Res* 1996; 11:1185-1190.

Cofrancesco J, Dobs AS. Transdermal testosterone delivery systems. *Endocrinologist* 1996; 6:207-213.

Jackson J, Kleerekoper M. Osteoporosis in men: diagnosis, pathophysiology, and prevention. *Medicine* 1990; 69(3):137-152.

Nguyen, TV et al. Risk factors for osteoporotic fractures in elderly men. *Am J Epidemiol* 1996; 144:255-263.

Seeman E et al. Risk factors for osteoporosis in men. *Am J Med* 1983; 75:977-983.

Warhaftig N et al. Determinants of bone mineral density in older men. *J Bone Miner Res* 1995; 10(11):1769-77.

CALCIUM QUESTIONAIRE

Estimate the calcium for each food you had for 1 week, and write it in the appropriate column. At the end of the week, add up the total calcium for each food. Add all the totals in the "total" column and divide that number by 7. This will give you an estimate of daily calcium. Consult the table on page 89 to find out if your calcium intake is sufficient.

FOOD	CALCIUIM	MON	TUES	WED	THU	FRI	SAT	SUN	TOTAL
MILK									
Milk (skim, 2%, whole), 1 c	300 mg								
Chocolate, 1 cup	280 mg								
Condensed, sweetened, 1 c	802 mg								
Evaporated, 1 cup	635 mg								
Powdered, 1/4 cup	200 mg								
YOGURT									
Plain, lowfat, 1 cup*	415 mg								
Plain, nonfat, 1 cup*	452 mg								
Low fat, fruit, 1 cup*	343 mg								
Yogurt cheese, 1 cup	550 mg								
CHEESE									
American, Velveeta, 1 oz	162 mg								
Blue, Romano, 1 oz	155 mg								
Brick, cheddar, edam, gouda, monterey jack, mozzarella, muenster, provolone, 1 oz	200 mg								
Brie, 1 oz	52 mg								
Camembert, 1 oz	30 mg								
Cottage cheese, 1/2 cup	69 mg								
Feta, 1 oz	100 mg								
Parmesan, 1 Tbsp	70 mg								
Ricotta (part-skim), 1 oz	84 mg								
Ricotta (whole), 1 oz	65 mg								
Swiss, 1 oz	272 mg								
SEAFOOD									
Clams, 1 cup (canned)	121 mg								
Makerel, 1 cup (canned)	552 mg								
Oysters, raw, 1 cup	226 mg								
Sardines & bones, 3 oz (can)	372 mg								
Salmon & bones, 3 oz (can)	200 mg								
Shrimp, 1 cup	147 mg								

* with added milk solids

FOOD	CALCIUIM	MON	TUES	WED	THU	FRI	SAT	SUN	TOTAL
VEGETABLES (1 CUP COOKED)									
Broccoli	178 mg								
Bok choy	250 mg								
Collard greens	299 mg								
Kale or mustard greens	157 mg								
Spinach or turnip greens	196 mg								
Swiss chard	148 mg								
Beans, all types	80 mg								
SWEETS AND NUTS (1 CUP)									
Ice cream (hard)	194 mg								
Ice cream (soft)	236 mg								
Ice milk (hard)	204 mg								
Ice milk (soft)	274 mg								
Frozen yogurt	160 mg								
Pudding (instant)	374 mg								
Pudding (cooked)	265 mg								
Custard (baked)	297 mg								
Almonds, chopped	304 mg								
Pecans, chopped	86 mg								
Peanuts or walnuts, chop.	100 mg								
MISCELLANEOUS									
Cream soup, with milk, 1 c	184 mg								
Frozen pizza, 4.5" arc	89 mg								
Carob flour, 1 cup	480 mg								
Blackstrap molasses, 1 Tbs	137 mg								
Tofu, set with calcium, 1/2 c	258 mg								
Soybeans, sprouted, 1 cup	54 mg								
Sunflower seeds, 1 cup	174 mg								
CALCIUM-FORTIFIED FOODS									
Calci-Milk, 1 cup	500 mg								
Citrus Hill orange juice, 1 c	300 mg								
Minute Maid orange juice, 1 c	320 mg								
Tropicana orange juice, 1 c	333 mg								
Total cereal, 3/4 cup	250 mg								
Wonder Bread, 2 slices	580 mg								

Index

Your bones can get stronger
if you know what to do

√ *Stand Tall! Every Woman's Guide to Preventing and Treating Osteo-porosis.* A caring gift for those you love.

√ *Osteoporosis: There IS Something You Can Do About It!*
     by Sara Meeks, P.T., G.C.S.
This is a comprehensive program for postural correction and back-strengthening. Helpful for postural problems or back pain, essential if you have low bone mass; straightens up a stooped back for many people. Includes a Thera-Band®, to be used for the resistive exercise portion of the program.

√ *Not Just Cheesecake! A Yogurt Cheese Cookbook (2nd ed.)*
     by Shelley Melvin
250 delicious high-calcium recipes (86 are low-calorie desserts!), with nutritional information and exchanges. All natural, no additives, easy to make.

√ *Mike's Famous Yogurt Cheese Maker*
The easy way to make low-fat or non-fat yogurt cheese—to boost calcium as well as lose weight, cut cholesterol and lower sodium. Enjoy plain or in recipes instead of cream cheese, whipped cream or sour cream.

√ *Save Your Bones! High Calcium, Low Calorie Recipes for the Family*
     by Lois Goulder
75 delicious, easy-to-make recipes, with shopping guide and sample menus. Appetizers, soups, salads, entrees, vegetables, desserts.

     For information about any of the above,
     write to Triad at P.O. Box 13355,
     Gainesville, FL 32604, or fax your
     questions to 1-800-854-4947.

√ *National Osteoporosis Foundation's* quarterly Newletter can help you stay up-to-date on new developments. For information, contact NOF directly at 1150 17th Street, NW, Suite 500, Washington, DC 20036, or call (202) 223-2226.